Oculoplasty for Ophthalmologists

Essam A. El Toukhy

Editor

Oculoplasty
for Ophthalmologists

Questions and Answers

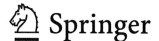 Springer

Editor
Essam A. El Toukhy
Oculoplasty Service
Cairo University
Cairo, Egypt

ISBN 978-3-030-68468-6   ISBN 978-3-030-68469-3   (eBook)
https://doi.org/10.1007/978-3-030-68469-3

This Springer imprint is published by the registered company Springer Nature Switzerland AG
The registered company address is: Gewerbestrasse 11, 6330 Cham, Switzerland

Preface

This book presents the most up-to-date oculoplastic knowledge base in a question and answer format. Multiple choice questions are the most commonly used assessment and teaching technique, and this question format will continue to assume a greater significance in the era of online exams and virtual consultations.

This book is designed to target ophthalmologists at varying professional levels; from residents and fellows to consultants. Whether they are preparing for an exam, sitting for a final degree, pursuing subspecialty training in oculoplasty, or requiring a detailed knowledge base of the subspecialty as they encounter clinical cases, this book provides a comprehensive guide from the very basic principles to the most advanced. The book will also be of special interest for consultant ophthalmologists and university professors organizing and preparing exams.

The book follows the same structure of the accompanying textbook "Oculoplastic Surgery—A Practical Guide to Common Disorders." Section by section, it includes over 1000 classic multiple choice questions as well as 150 high-quality clinical photos and illustrations with a variety of case presentations, clinical scenarios, radiological scans, and pathological specimens. The questions are meant to supplement the information provided in the textbook, which is available for further clarification and in-depth study of the various subjects. This supplementary approach and extensive illustrative support makes this book series unique in the world of oculoplasty (at present, no high-quality referenced question books are available at international level).

We hope this book becomes a staple on every ophthalmologist's desk as they pursue the specialty and encounter oculoplasty cases in their practice.

Cairo, Egypt   Essam A. El Toukhy

Acknowledgements   To all those who supported me during my life, to all the wonderful people in my life, my dear parents, my lovely wife, and my beloved daughters.

Contents

Basics of Oculoplasty and Anaesthesia

Essam A. El Toukhy

Oculoplastic surgery is the subspecialty that combines the art and principles of plastic and reconstructive surgery with the delicacy and precision of ophthalmic surgery. An oculoplastic surgeon should be aware of the principles of both worlds as well as surgical skills to get optimum cosmetic and functional results while protecting the globe and the patient's vision. A thorough knowledge of wound healing, the types of sutures, needles, flaps and grafts is mandatory to gain a cosmetically accepted result.

Similarly, anaesthesia is an indispensable component of Oculoplastic procedures. As a subspecialty, oculoplasty has its own needs and requirements regarding anaesthesia management, with tailored approaches of local, regional and general anaesthesia techniques. Anaesthetic management for oculoplastic surgeries mainly requires a thorough knowledge of the anatomy as well as local anaesthetic pharmacology. Regional blocks have gained widespread enthusiasm and are being used more and more frequently now. They can be used alone or in combination with each other to cover the surgery site. They cause minimal discomfort, lower cost, and lower perioperative morbidity in comparison to general anaesthesia. They also provide the advantages of less local anaesthetic use and minimal tissue distortion when compared with infiltration anaesthesia.

E. A. El Toukhy (✉)
Oculoplasty Service, Cairo University, Cairo, Egypt
e-mail: eeltoukhy@yahoo.com

Basics of Oculoplasty and Anaesthesia

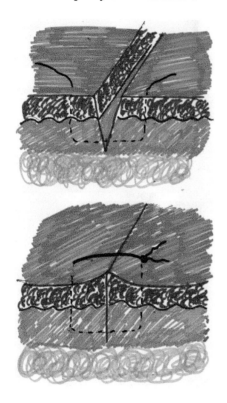

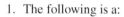

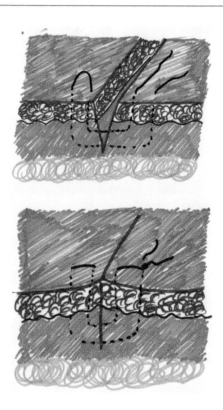

2. The following is a:

   A. Vertical mattress suture
   B. Horizontal mattress suture
   C. Interrupted suture
   D. Continuous suture.

1. The following is a:

   A. Vertical mattress suture
   B. Horizontal mattress suture
   C. Interrupted suture
   D. Continuous suture.

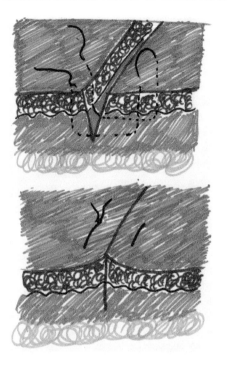

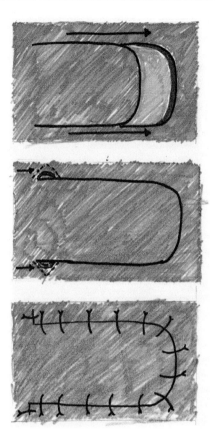

3. The following is a:

   A. Vertical mattress suture
   B. Horizontal mattress suture
   C. Interrupted suture
   D. Continuous suture.

4. The above diagram is an example of:

   A. Advancing flap
   B. Rotational flap
   C. Rhomboid flap
   D. Transpositional flap.

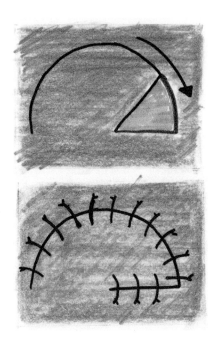

6. The above diagram is an example of:

   A. Advancing flap
   B. Rotational flap
   C. Rhomboid flap
   D. Transpositional flap.

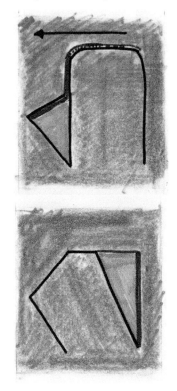

5. The above diagram is an example of:

   A. Advancing flap
   B. Rotational flap
   C. Rhomboid flap
   D. Transpositional flap.

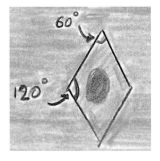

7. The above diagram is an example of:

   A. Advancing flap
   B. Rotational flap
   C. Rhomboid flap
   D. Transpositional flap.

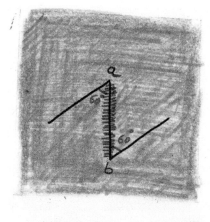

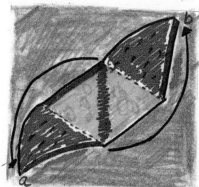

8. The following technique can be useful in the management of all except:

   A. Scar revision
   B. Cicatricial ectropion
   C. Cicatricial entropion
   D. Eyelid Webbing.

9. The following are true EXCEPT:

   A. The supraorbital ridge extends only over the medial one half to two thirds of the superior orbital rim
   B. The frontalis muscle of the forehead supports medial two thirds of the eyebrow
   C. The sensory nerves to the forehead travel on the underside of the frontalis
   D. The supratrochlear nerve supplies most of the sensation of the forehead.

10. The following are true about the nasociliary nerve EXCEPT:

   A. Gives off supratrochlear nerve which innervates the medial forehead
   B. It supplies the lateral wall of the nose
   C. Innervates the cornea
   D. Carries within it the sympathetic fibers from the internal carotid plexus.

11. The long ciliary nerve:

   A. Enters the globe at the equator
   B. Contains parasympathetic nerve fibres
   C. Synapse at the ciliary ganglion
   D. Contains sensory fibres from the cornea.

12. The following is TRUE about the superior ophthalmic vein:

   A. It is the main venous channel of the orbit
   B. It is formed by the union between the facial vein and the temporal vein
   C. It passes backward in the orbit between the levator and the superior rectus muscle
   D. It does not receive the central retinal vein.

13. The peripheral arterial arcade in the upper eyelid is present:

   A. 3 mm above the eyelid margin
   B. Along the anterior surface of the tarsus
   C. Between the levator aponeurosis and Muller's muscle
   D. Between the orbicularis oculi muscle and levator aponeurosis.

14. All of the following structures attach to the Whitnal's tubercle except

   A. Superior transverse ligament of the orbit
   B. Aponeurosis of the levator palpebrae superioris muscle
   C. Suspensory ligament of the eyeball
   D. Lateral check ligament of the inferior oblique muscle.

15. All of the following structures pass through the superior orbital fissure, except

   A. Sympathetic nerve fibers
   B. Superior ophthalmic vein
   C. Trochlear nerve
   D. Zygomatic nerve.

16. What tissue plane is the temporal branch of the facial nerve located in, superior to the zygomatic arch?

    A. Deep temporal fascia
    B. Loose areolar tissue
    C. Subcutaneous tissue
    D. Temporoparietal fascia.

17. The gray line of the eyelid margin is formed by

    A. Meibomian glands
    B. Tarsal border
    C. Mucocutaneous junction
    D. Orbicularis muscle.

18. The capsulopalpebral fascia is analogous to which upper eyelid structure?

    A. Levator aponeurosis
    B. Orbital septum
    C. Superior transverse ligament
    D. Muller's muscle.

19. The normal horizontal measurement of the palpebral fissure is approximately

    A. 20 mm
    B. 25 mm
    C. 30 mm
    D. 35 mm.

20. Which statement about the orbital septum is *false*?

    A. During entropion repair, it is very important to recognize the orbital septum of the lower eyelid as being different from the aponeurosis or lower eyelid retractors
    B. The orbital septum arises from a condensation of the periosteum of the orbital rim called the *arcus marginalis*
    C. The orbital septum inserts on the superior border of the tarsus in the upper eyelid
    D. The orbital septum serves as a barrier to the spread of infection from the superficial eyelids to the orbital tissues.

21. Which statement concerning the medial canthal area is *true*?

    A. All of the attachments anchoring the tarsi to the medial orbital wall lie anterior to the lacrimal sac and attach to the maxillary portion of the frontal bone
    B. The lacrimal sac lies posterior to the orbital septum
    C. The muscle pump of the lacrimal pump mechanism is innervated by the fifth cranial nerve
    D. Lockwood ligament attaches posterior to the lacrimal sac.

22. Which statement regarding fat encountered during eyelid surgery is *false*?

    A. Preaponeurotic fat is orbital fat
    B. Extraconal orbital fat is an important landmark in identifying the levator aponeurosis
    C. The removal of fat from the upper eyelid nasal, central, and lateral fat pads may be done with impunity
    D. In the upper eyelid, the nasal fat pad is small, whereas the lateral fat pad is the small fat pad in the lower eyelid.

23. Which statement regarding Whitnall ligament (superior transverse ligament) is *false*?

    A. Whitnall ligament attaches medially to the trochlea, laterally to the capsule of the lacrimal gland, and to the lateral orbital wall
    B. This ligament is a condensation of the sheath of the levator muscle and serves as a check ligament to prevent excessive elevation of the eyelid
    C. Whitnall ligament acts to change the direction of pull of the levator muscle from horizontal to vertical
    D. This ligament passes anterior to the lacrimal gland.

24. Which statement about eyelid anatomy is *false*?

    A. The gray line is formed by the muscle of Riolan and represents the observable edge of the pretarsal orbicularis at the eyelid margin
    B. The posterior lamella of the eyelid consists of the conjunctiva and tarsus
    C. The mucocutaneous junction occurs where the eyelashes emerge from the eyelid
    D. The peripheral and marginal arterial arcades allow for anastomosis between the internal and external carotid systems.

25. Features of the orbicularis muscle include:

    A. Closure of the eyelid, depression of the eyebrow, and facilitation of tear drainage
    B. Pretarsal orbicularis inserts temporally to become the lateral canthal tendon, ontraction narrows the palpebral fissure, and the orbital portion of the muscle inserts medially on the posterior lacrimal crest
    C. The deep head of the medial pretarsal muscle is called *Homer tensor tarsi* and innervation of the orbicularis muscle by cranial nerve III is divided into three segments (pretarsal, preseptal, and orbital)
    D. The zygomaticofacial nerve innervates the upper lid orbicularis, the frontal branch of cranial nerve VII sends motor fibers to the upper lid orbicularis, and the preseptal orbicularis divides to encompass the lacrimal gland.

26. Which one of the following muscle groups is paired *incorrectly*?

    A. Tensor tarsi muscle-deep head of the pretarsal orbicularis
    B. Nasalis-preseptal orbicularis
    C. Superciliary corrugator muscle-orbital orbicularis
    D. Frontalis-procerus muscle.

27. Which structure and its bony framework are paired *incorrectly*?

    A. Lacrimal sac fossa-lacrimal and maxillary bones
    B. Optic canal-greater and lesser wings of the sphenoid bone
    C. Inferior orbital fissure-maxilla, zygomatic bone, palatine bone, and greater wing of the sphenoid bone
    D. Anterior and posterior ethmoidal foramen-ethmoid and frontal bones.

28. All of the following statements concerning lymphatic and venous drainage are true *except*:

    A. Lymphatic vessels of the orbit drain along the lateral portion of the cavernous sinus
    B. Lymphatic vessels serving the medial portion of the upper eyelid drain into submandibular lymph nodes
    C. Lymphatic vessels serving the lateral portions of the upper eyelid drain into preauricular nodes
    D. Pretarsal venous drainage of the medial upper eyelid is into the angular vein and the lateral venous drainage is into the superficial temporal vein system.

29. Regarding the orbital septum, which is incorrect:

    A. Is separated from the levator aponeurosis by orbital fat
    B. Is firmly attached to Whitnall's ligament
    C. Fuses with the capsulopalpebral fascia in the lower lid
    D. Inserts on the levator aponeurosis about 3 to 5 mm above the tarsal plate.

30. Regarding the tarsal plates, which is incorrect:

    A. Of the upper lid are about 10 mm in height
    B. Of the lower lid are about 8 mm in height
    C. Impart structural integrity to the eyelids
    D. Do not contain lash follicles.

31. Regarding the orbital floor is, which is incorrect:

    A. Composed primarily of the maxillary bone
    B. Composed of the zygomatic and palatine bones
    C. Separated from the lateral wall by the inferior orbital fissure
    D. The largest of the orbital walls, running to the orbital apex.

32. Regarding the medial orbital wall, which is incorrect:

    A. Contains the frontal process of the maxillary bone
    B. Contains the optic foramen
    C. Is composed of the sphenoid bone and the lacrimal bone.
    D. Is composed largely of the ethmoid bone.

33. Regarding the ophthalmic artery, which is incorrect:

    A. Crosses over the optic nerve in 85% of individuals
    B. Enters the orbit through the optic canal
    C. Gives off the lacrimal artery as its first orbital branch
    D. Gives off the central retinal artery which runs under the optic nerve.

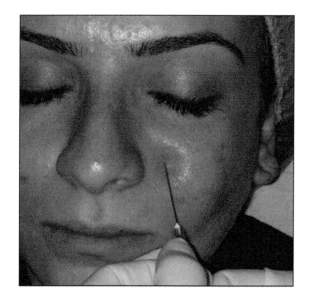

34. The above nerve block is indicated in surgeries on all except:

    A. Lower eyelid
    B. Lower canaliculus
    C. DCR
    D. Lower lid entropion.

35. Malignant hyperthermia occurs mostly in all except:

    A. Children
    B. Adults
    C. Ptosis
    D. Strabismus.

36. Lidocaine is:

    A. An amide anesthetic
    B. Has a rapid onset of action
    C. Is an intermediate acting drug
    D. Has low systemic toxicity.

37. Phantom eye syndrome can be prevented by:

    A. General anesthesia
    B. Performing evisceration rather than enucleation
    C. Removing a long stump of the optic nerve
    D. Insertion of an orbital implant.

38. All the following are phases of wound healing except:

A. Inflammatory phase
B. Scarring phase
C. Proliferation phase
D. Remodeling phase.

39. Scar formation is influenced by all except:

A. Site
B. Age
C. Sex
D. Skin type.

40. A bad scar can be due to all except:

A. Smoking
B. Poor surgical technique
C. Wound tension
D. Undermining of surrounding tissues.

41. Monofilament sutures are preferable in:

A. Tarsal suturing
B. Muscle suturing
C. Skin suturing
D. Tendon suturing.

42. 1/2 circle needles are used in

A. Skin closure to reduce scarring
B. Ptosis surgery to suture the levator aponeurosis to the tarsus
C. DCR surgery for closure of the posterior flaps
D. Brow pexy procedures.

43. Graft "take" means occurrence of:

A. Fibroblast proliferation
B. Fibrin deposition
C. Vascularization
D. Neurotization.

44. In lid reconstruction; one can use all except:

A. A flap for the anterior lamella and a flap for the posterior lamella
B. A flap for the anterior lamella and a graft for the posterior lamella
C. A graft for the anterior lamella and a flap for the posterior lamella
D. A graft for the anterior lamella and a graft for the posterior lamella.

45. Pain during local anesthesia injection can be reduced by;

A. Slow injection
B. Smaller needles
C. Addition of bicarbonate
D. Needle-free jet injections.

46. Disadvantages of local infiltration anesthesia during ptosis surgery include all except:

A. Hematoma formation
B. Stimulation of Muller muscle by epinephrine
C. Diffusion of the anesthetic to orbicularis muscle
D. Diffusion of the anesthetic to the levator muscle.

47. Reflex sneezing while injecting local anesthesia (sternutatory reflex) is mediated by:

A. Infraorbital nerve
B. Supraorbital nerve
C. Nasociliary nerve
D. Lacrimal nerve.

Answers of Basics of Oculoplasty and Anaesthesia

1	C	13	C	25	A	37	B
2	A	14	D	26	B	38	B
3	B	15	D	27	B	39	C
4	A	16	D	28	A	40	D
5	B	17	D	29	B	41	C
6	C	18	A	30	B	42	C
7	D	19	C	31	D	43	C
8	C	20	C	32	B	44	D
9	D	21	D	33	C	45	D
10	A	22	C	34	D	46	C
11	D	23	D	35	B	47	C
12	A	24	C	36	D		

Lid Lesions and Malpositions

2

Essam A. El Toukhy

Introduction

Various lesions can be detected in the eyelid due to its diverse composition. The skin epidermis is keratinized stratified squamous epithelium while its dermis contains cilia in addition to modified sweat and sebaceous glands. The tarsus also contains Meibomian glands which are modified sebaceous glands while the lining conjunctiva contains accessory lacrimal glands and goblet cells.

Skin adnexa including sebaceous and sweat glands as well as hair follicles are placed in the dermis and can give an origin to a wide variety of, usually, benign lesions.

The sebaceous glands of the eye lid include; the Meibomian gland of the tarsus, glands of Zeis that are related to the eye lashes and the sebaceous glands related to hair of the eyelid skin as well as the hair of the eye brow.

The sweat glands of the eyelid are either eccrine glands (that have a true secretory duct) that are present everywhere in the body skin including the eyelid or apocrine glands (that have no duct and secrete by cellular decapitation) that are present in relation to eyelashes and known as glands of Moll.

The majority of the lid lesions are benign, but their identification is important for proper treatment and to rule out malignancy.

The main goal of the ophthalmologist is to exclude malignancy. Certain points in history taking and clinical examination help to rule out malignant lesions.

Benign lesions are usually uniform with regular borders and show slow growth. They usually don't show induration, ulceration or lid margin destruction and can be classified according to;

- Structure of origin to epidermal, dermal or adnexal.
- Clinical appearance either solid or cystic.
- Location whither related to the lid margin, pretarsal area or supra/infra tarsal region.

On the other hand, features suspicious of malignancy include:

- Recent onset.
- Increasing in size.
- Change in color or multiple colors.
- Ulceration.
- Telangiectasia.
- Pearly borders.
- Ill-defined margins.
- Distorted anatomy e.g. loss of lashes, distorted lid margin.
- Recurrent lesion e.g. recurrent chalazion.

E. A. El Toukhy (✉)
Oculoplasty Service, Cairo University, Cairo, Egypt
e-mail: eeltoukhy@yahoo.com

© The Author(s), under exclusive license to Springer Nature Switzerland AG 2021
E. A. El Toukhy (ed.), *Oculoplasty for Ophthalmologists*, https://doi.org/10.1007/978-3-030-68469-3_2

- Pain disproportional to the lesion i.e. perineural spread.
- History of irradiation e.g. for acne, retinoblastoma.
- History of other malignancies.
- Immunosuppression.

Generally, the clinical appearance is highly suggestive of the lesion nature yet, when in doubt, a biopsy is required to confirm the diagnosis. Biopsies are either incisional which entails removal of a part of the lesion or excisional in which the lesion is totally removed thus, additionally provides a cure.

Treatment options in general include total excision of the lesion, with special attention to removal of the walls in case of cysts, marsupialization i.e. removal of the top of the cyst if excision is not feasible and surface ablation in superficial lesions.

The goals of therapy for periocular lid malignancy are threefold: to completely excise the tumor; to maintain the integrity and the function of the eye; and to achieve a good cosmetic result.

It may be difficult to accomplish all of these objectives in every patient or by one surgery. The dilemma of removal of the tumor while preserving normal tissue is more challenging in the periocular area than it is on other areas on the skin.

Lid reconstruction should aim at restoration of normal lid anatomy with replacement of defect in the anterior and/or posterior lamella using the appropriate reconstructive surgical technique, individualized for each case.

Radiotherapy, Photodynamic therapy, cryotherapy, Topical immunotherapy, topical and systemic chemotherapy can all be used as an adjuvant, or instead of, surgical excision in some cases.

The eyelids are the primary defense of the eye against dryness, exposure, and trauma. Therefore, proper lid positioning is important to ocular health. Lid malpositions are among the most common problems encountered by the ophthalmologist. Visual loss may occur in these conditions due to keratopathy secondary to exposure or lashes rubbing on the ocular surface.

A thorough understanding of the anatomy, pathophysiology, appropriate evaluation, and treatment options of these lid malpositions is essential for the practicing ophthalmologist.

The classification of lid malpositions is based according to their respective etiologies. There are five main types of ectropion: involutional, paralytic, mechanical, cicatricial, and congenital. Entropion is subdivided into 4 categories: involutional, acute spastic, cicatricial, and congenital. Facial nerve affection can result in more than one type of lid malpositions. Lid retraction, Centurion syndrome, Floppy eyelids syndrome are less common lid malpositions seen in clinical practice.

The preoperative evaluation is essential for determining the etiology of the lid malposition and deciding on the surgical procedure necessary for correction of the malposition.

The goal of a successful surgical repair includes a good apposition of the lid margin to the globe, corneal irritation symptoms relief, good cosmetic outcome with lasting results, while addressing the underlying pathophysiology.

Being the most common cause of infectious blindness and a leading cause of lid lesions and malpositions globally, trachoma deserves a special emphasis.

Lid Lesions

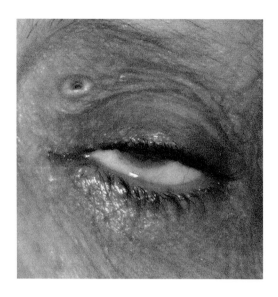

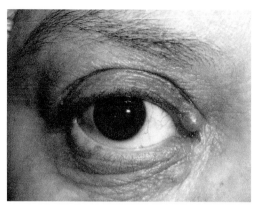

3. The above figure is
    A. Cyst of Moll
    B. Molluscum contagiousum
    C. Hidrocystoma
    D. Keratoacanthoma.

1. The above figure is
    A. Sebaceous cyst
    B. Molluscum contagiousum
    C. Nevus
    D. Keratoacanthoma.

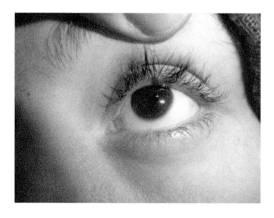

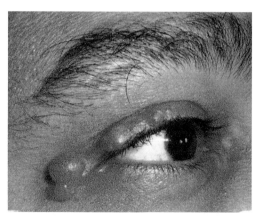

4. The above figure is
    A. Cyst of Moll
    B. Molluscum contagiousum
    C. Hidrocystoma
    D. Keratoacanthoma.

2. The above figure is;
    A. Junctional nevus
    B. Compound nevus
    C. Congenital nevus
    D. Kissing nevus.

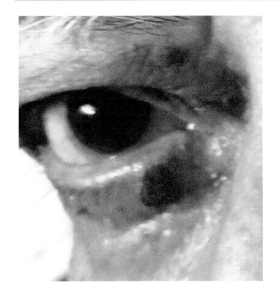

5. The above figure is
    A. Sebaceous cyst
    B. Molluscum contagiousum
    C. Seborrheic keratosis
    D. Keratoacanthoma.

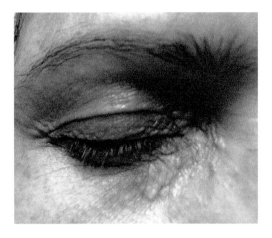

6. The above lesion is best treated by:
    A. Observation
    B. Radiofrequenc
    C. Laser
    D. Surgery.

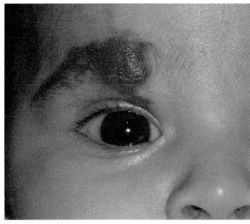

7. The above lesion can be treated by all
    except:
    A. Observation
    B. Steroids
    C. B blocker
    D. Surgery.

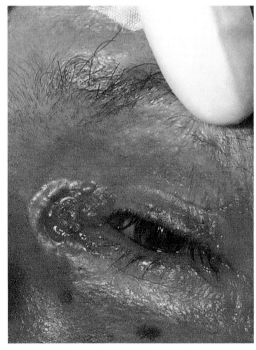

8. The most likely diagnosis of the above lesion is:
   A. Sebaceous cell carcinoma
   B. Basal cell carcinoma
   C. Squamous cell carcinoma
   D. Amelanotic malignant melanoma.

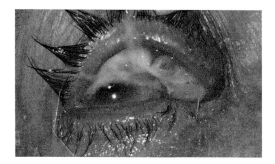

9. The most likely diagnosis of the above lesion is:
   A. Sebaceous cell carcinoma
   B. Basal cell carcinoma
   C. Squamous cell carcinoma
   D. Amelanotic malignant melanoma.

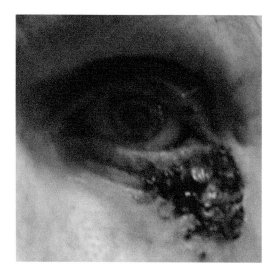

10. The most likely diagnosis of the above lesion is:
    A. Sebaceous cell carcinoma
    B. Basal cell carcinoma
    C. Squamous cell carcinoma
    D. Amelanotic malignant melanoma.

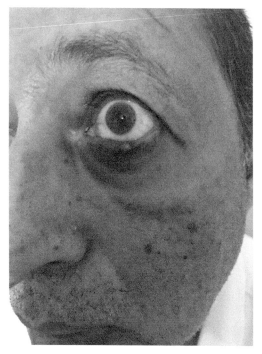

11. Features suggesting malignancy in this lesion include all except:
    A. Loss of lashes
    B. Short history
    C. Recurrence after previous excision
    D. Telangiectacic vessels.

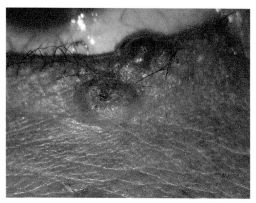

12. The likely diagnosis of the above lesion includes all except:
    A. Pigmented Sebaceous cell carcinoma
    B. Pigmented Basal cell carcinoma
    C. Pigmented Squamous cell carcinoma
    D. Malignant melanoma.

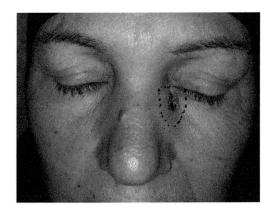

13. Management of the lacrimal drainage system in this patient with a malignant lid lesion in a young patient is:
    A. Preservation of the lower canaliculus
    B. Excision of the lower canaliculus without intubation
    C. Excision of the lower canaliculus with intubation
    D. Excision of the lower canaliculus with placement of Jones tube.

14. The Breslow scale:
    A. Is a measurement of the thickness of cutaneous malignant melanoma
    B. Highly correlates with prognosis
    C. The prognosis is poor if more than 2 mm
    D. Is incorporated in the TNM staging.

15. The Clark scale:
    A. Is a histopathological scale used to grade malignant melanoma
    B. Depends on the level of invasion of the tumor cells
    C. The higher the scale, the worse the prognosis
    D. Is incorporated in the TNM staging.

16. The treatment of choice for keratocanthoma is:
    A. Observation
    B. Steroid injection
    C. Incisional biopsy followed by complete surgical excision
    D. Cryotherapy.

17. In treatment of chalazion:
    A In the acute phase topical antibiotics is recommended
    B. Systemic doxycycline is used in acute secondary infection for short time
    C. Surgical incision for chronic cystic chalazion is recommend
    D. Histopathology is performed on excised chalazion for the possibility of malignant transformation of chalazion.

18. One of the following signs suggest eyelid malignancy:
    A. Superficial vascularization
    B. Hypopigmentation
    C. Painful lesions
    D. Fast growing.

19. Regarding lid pigmentary lesions, the most appropriate statement is:
    A. Nevi are the least common
    B. Freckle are result of hyperpigmentation of the basal layer of epidermis
    C. Malignant transformation is common with compound nevi
    D. Blue nevus has no potential malignant transformation.

20. The most common precancerous lesion is:
    A. Solar lentigo
    B. Dermal melanocytosis
    C. Actinic keratosis
    D. Keratoacanthoma.

21. A 52 years old white male presenting with lower lid ulcerating lesion near the medial canthus. Family history is positive for xeroderma pigmentosa. The most likely diagnosis of this lesion is:
    A. Squamous cell carcinoma
    B. Basal cell carcinoma
    C. Melanoma
    D. Sebaceous cell carcinoma.

22. In patients with Bowen disease:
    A. Histopathology shows limitation of the disease to dermal layer of the skin

B. Cryotherapy is good treatment modality for the skin lesions

C. 50% can progress to squamous cell carcinoma

D. Skin lesions are rapidly increasing in size.

23. Regarding keratoacanthoma one of the following statement is true:
   A. Considered a benign lesion
   B. Rapidly progressing in size
   C. Typically occurs in young adults
   D. Excisional biopsy is not required.

24. Regarding basal cell nevus syndrome (Gorlin-Goltz syndrome), which is incorrect:
   A. Is inherited as an autosomal dominant trait
   B. Includes jaw cysts
   C. Includes mental retardation
   D. Generally appears before age 10 years.

25. The least appropriate statement regarding basal cell carcinoma is:
   A. Head and neck account for 90% of cases
   B. 10% of head and neck cases involve eyelids
   C. Usually adults between 50-80 years of age
   D. 15% of eyelid cases in patients under 35 years.

26. The least likely Indications for removing nevus is:
   A. Acquired lesion
   B. Congenital lesion
   C. Irritation induced area
   D. Sun exposed area.

27. Regarding sebaceous adenocarcinoma:
   A. It can arise from eyelid skin sebaceous glands
   B. More common in males
   C. Lower lid is more frequently involved
   D. Regional lymph nodes involvement is sentinel lymph node biopsy is not recommended.

28. A 45 year old man presents with rapidly enlarging mass below the eyelid margin the lesion has a central crater with an elevated rolled edge. The most likely diagnosis is:
   A. Epidermal inclusion cyst
   B. Keratoacanthoma
   C. Verruca vulgaris
   D. Pilomatricoma.

29. Apocrine hidrocystoma is
   A. Considered a true adenoma
   B. Deep cyst requires marsupialization
   C. It's also known as cylindromas
   D. Histopathologically it is squamous cystic structure containing keratin.

30. A 70-year-old patient presents with a history of a painless, progressively enlarging mass in the central aspect of the right upper lid. On examination, there is some distortion of the eyelid margin and loss of lashes. The most likely diagnosis is:
   A. Basal cell carcinoma
   B. Sebaceous gland carcinoma
   C. Squamous cell carcinoma
   D. Amelanotic melanoma.

31. Squamous cell carcinoma of the eyelid, one is false:
   A. It is 40 times less common than basal cell carcinoma
   B. It is more aggressive than basal cell carcinoma
   C. Surgical excision with wide margin is preferred
   D. Only metastasize through blood borne transmission.

32. Which of the following pairs of eyelid lesions and their histological features is FALSE?
   A. Basal cell carcinoma—peripheral palisading nuclei
   B. Squamous cell carcinoma—keratin pearls
   C. Keratoacanthoma—hypokeratosis
   D. Sebaceous cell carcinoma—pagetoid spread.

33. Which of the following eyelid tumors is NOT an indication for sentinel lymph node biopsy?
    A. Sebaceous cell carcinoma
    B. Malignant melanoma
    C. Basal cell carcinoma
    D. Squamous cell carcinoma.

34. A 60 years old patient presented with large upper lid lesion of 6 months duration, lid margin irregularities was seen with loss of eyelashes overlying the lesion.The best next step will be;
    A. Excision and drainage of the chalazion
    B. Initial treatment with topical antibiotics
    C. Excisional biopsy
    D. Orbital CT.

35. All of the followings are correct for squamous cell carcinoma of the eyelids except:
    A. Is more common in the lightly pigmented individuals than in highly pigmented ones
    B. May occur in scar tissue of highly pigmented individuals
    C. Does not arise from actinic lesions
    D. Is associated with psoralen plus UV-A light therapy for psoriasis.

36. What is the sebaceous cell carcinoma's response to radiation therapy?
    A. Very susceptible when used as an adjunct to surgery
    B. Responsive when combined with photodynamic agents
    C. Relatively radio-resistant
    D. Needs multiple sessions.

37. Which one of the following is NOT a feature of basal cell carcinoma?
    A. Pearly elevated margins
    B. Spread to regional lymph nodes
    C. Ulcerated epithelium
    D. Telangiectatic vessels.

38. In treatment of chalazion:
    A. In the acute phase topical antibiotics are recommended

B. Systemic doxycycline is used in acute secondary infection for short time
C. Surgical incision for a chronic cystic chalazion is recommended
D. A horizontal incision is recommended.

39. An elderly female presented with recurrent swelling of the upper eyelid. Histopathological evaluation revealed it to be a chalazion. What would be the histopathological finding?
    A. Lipogranuloma
    B. Suppurative granuloma
    C. Foreign body granuloma
    D. Xanthogranuloma.

40. All of the following are true regarding chalazion, except:
    A. Sebaceous cyst
    B. It is due to staphylococcal infection
    C. Recurrence may imply malignancy
    D. Occlusion of the meibomian gland.

41. Treatment of chalazion includes:
    A. Incision and drainage
    B. Intralesional steroid
    C. Pressure bandage
    D. Antibiotics.

42. A recurrent chalazion should be subjected to histopathological examination to rule out the possibility of
    A. Squamous cell carcinoma
    B. Sebaceous cell carcinoma
    C. Malignant melanoma
    D. Basal cell carcinoma.

43. All of the following are true about BCC, except:
    A. Spread to the regional lymph nodes occurs late
    B. Occurs more frequently in immunosuppressed individuals
    C. Complete surgical excision is advised
    D. The lesion may involute over several months.

44. What is the most appropriate initial step in the management of a suspicious lesion on the lid margin of a 50 years old male?
    A. Incision and curettage
    B. Observation
    C. Full-thickness excisional biopsy
    D. Incisional biopsy.

45. Which of the following papillomatous lesions of the eyelid is premalignant?
    A. Acanthosis nigricans
    B. Actinic keratosis
    C. Seborrheic keratosis
    D. Verruca vulgaris.

46. Which of the following papillomatous lesions of the eyelid may be associated with underlying systemic malignancy?
    A. Acanthosis nigricans
    B. Verruca vulgaris
    C. Ephelis
    D. Actinic keratosis.

47. All of the following are true regarding sebaceous carcinoma, except:
    A. The primary focus may be either eyelid or caruncle
    B. Shave biopsy techniques are adequate
    C. The hallmarks of the histopathology of the condition include skip areas and pagetoid
    D. Recognition is often delayed due to misdiagnosis as benign eyelid inflammation.

48. All of the following are true regarding malignant melanoma of eyelid skin, except:
    A. Lentigo maligna melanoma and nodular melanoma are the most common forms affecting the eyelid
    B. Nodular melanoma has the worst prognosis
    C. The factor of greatest prognostic significance is depth of invasion
    D. Like conjunctival melanosis, eyelid melanoma may be controlled with cryotherapy.

49. A 14-years-old patient presents with a left upper eyelid lesion. Histopathology of the lesion showed shadow cells and areas of calcification surrounded by basophilic cells. All of the following are true of the patient's condition, except:
    A. Young adults are most often affected
    B. The lesion is epithelial in origin
    C. Surgical excision of the lesion is curative
    D. The eyebrow is also a common site of involvement.

50. A recurrent basal cell carcinoma extending deeply in the lateral orbit requires which treatment:
    A. Orbital exenteration
    B. Full-thickness pentagonal wedge resection
    C. Wide excision with cryotherapy
    D. Radiation therapy.

51. A patient with sebaceous carcinoma of the eyelid presents with an enlarged submandibular lymph node, which of the following is most likely to be the location of this patient's eyelid neoplasm?
    A. Medial, lower eyelid
    B. Lateral, lower eyelid
    C. Medial, upper eyelid
    D. Lateral, upper eyelid.

52. Which one of the following is a feature of basal cell carcinoma?
    A. Always has a predisposing precursor lesion
    B. Possible spread to regional lymph nodes
    C. Respects tissue planes
    D. Telangiectatic vessels.

53. The following factors are all associated with cutaneous cancers *except:*
    A. Increased sun exposure
    B. Increased age
    C. Red hair
    D. Increased natural skin pigmentation.

54. Features most consistent with a malignant eyelid lesion include:

A. Tenderness, erythema, alteration in pigment pattern
B. Disruption of tarsal architecture, raised pearly margins, pruritus
C. Lash loss, central ulceration, rapid growth
D. Ipsilateral lymph node metastasis, hyperkeratosis, dark pigmentation.

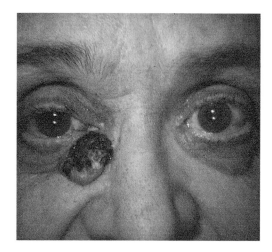

55. This lesion most likely represents:
A. Nodular basal cell carcinoma
B. Morpheaform basal cell carcinoma
C. Nodular squamous cell carcinoma
D. Sebaceous adenocarcinoma.

56. Features of a keratoacanthoma include all of the following *except*:
A. Spontaneous resolution
B. Loss of eyelashes
C. Ulcerated crater filled with lipids
D. Rapid growth.

57. Xanthelasma eyelid lesions have all the following features *except*:
A. Associated with systemic hyperlipidemic conditions in approximately 25% of patients
B. Located in the basal epithelial layer of the skin
C. Associated with the Erdheim-Chester disease

D. Microscopically contain foamy histiocytes.

58. Which of the following statements does not accurately describe a sebaceous cell adenocarcinoma lesion?
A. The lower eyelid is more frequently involved than the upper eyelid
B. Radiation therapy is thought to be a causative factor
C. Most arise from the meibomian glands of the tarsus
D. The initial course is indolent and often misdiagnosed.

59. Which of the following does not indicate a poor prognosis for a sebaceous cell adenocarcinoma lesion?
A. Duration of symptoms less than 6 months
B. Infiltrative growth pattern
C. Moderate or poor differentiation
D. Lymphatic or vascular invasion.

60. Chronic unilateral blepharoconjunctivitis is commonly a presenting sign of which one of the following?
A. Squamous cell carcinoma
B. Basal cell carcinoma
C. Cutaneous melanoma
D. Sebaceous carcinoma.

61. Which of the following statements most accurately describes the behavior and management of congenital nevi?
A. The risk of melanoma is directly related to the size of congenital nevi
B. Small congenital nevi do not need to be followed
C. Biopsy of congenital nevi is contraindicated
D. Large congenital nevi require complete surgical excision.

62. A patient presents with lentigo maligna involving the majority of the lower eyelid. What is the most appropriate management option?
A. Observation for thickening of the lesion
B. Radiation

C. Cryotherapy

D. Surgical excision with pathologic confirmation and delayed reconstruction.

63. Biopsy of a broad area of pigmentation of the eyelid has been read as lentigo maligna. What is the treatment of choice?
    A. Complete excision with adequate surgical margins
    B. Map biopsies looking for localized invasion
    C. Cryotherapy to the broad area
    D. Close observation.

64. Which of the following statements describes how to differentiate a compound from a junctional nevus?
    A. Compound nevi are larger
    B. Junctional nevi are darker and macular, or thinly papular, while compound nevi are lighter and elevated compared to uninvolved surrounding skin
    C. Junctional nevi show melanocytes in the superficial dermis
    D. Junctional nevi are more dome-shaped.

65. You have removed a medial canthal lesion which is diagnosed as basal cell carcinoma with morpheaform characteristics. The pathologist confirms the margins are negative in four quadrants (0°, 15°, 30°, 45°). What is the optimum next step?
    A. Adjunctive cryotherapy
    B. Excision with margin control because of the aggressive nature of the tumor
    C. Adjunctive alkylating agents
    D. Observation with return in one year.

66. Horizontal stability of the eyelid margin is essentially maintained by?
    A. Lid retractors
    B. Muscular tone
    C. Two point fixation
    D. Lid protractors.

67. A suspected upper eyelid chalazion in a 68-year-old patient demonstrates surrounding palpebral conjunctival inflammation,

raising concern about sebacaeous cell carcinoma. What is the optimum next step?
    A. Sentinal lymph node evaluation
    B. Full thickness biopsy and conjunctival map biopsies
    C. Shave biopsy
    D. Corticosteroid injection and curretage.

68. What is the role of cryotherapy in the treatment of eyelid melanoma?
    A. Possibly useful in conjunctival melanoma, but not in skin
    B. Recommended for both skin and conjunctiva
    C. Useful for skin, not conjunctiva
    D. Not useful for skin or conjunctiva.

69. What is the most important predicator for recurrence and survival in patients with eyelid melanocytic skin lesions?
    A. Excision margins
    B. Tumor thickness
    C. Diameter
    D. Geographic Location on eyelid.

70. For a basal-cell carcinoma of the eyelids, in what location is associated with the worst prognosis for recurrence and mortality?
    A. Lower eyelid margin
    B. Lower eyelid (not involving lid margin)
    C. Central upper eyelid
    D. Medial canthus.

71. What is the most common type of melanoma which occurs on the eyelids?
    A. Superficial spreading
    B. Nodular
    C. Acrolentiginous
    D. Lentigo maligna.

72. What clinical association is characteristic of lentigo maligna?
    A. It presents as a thickened and nodular pigmented mass
    B. It is characterized by rapid growth
    C. It may progress to lentigo maligna melanoma
    D. Premalignant changes are confined to the clinically involved area.

73. Regarding cutaneous horns, which is false:
    A. May develop from seborrheic keratosis
    B. May develop from basal cell carcinoma
    C. May develop from keratoacanthoma
    D. Should undergo biopsy.

74. Regarding keratoacanthoma, which is false:
    A. Usually develops over a period of weeks
    B. Does not exhibit cellular atypia
    C. May be associated with systemic malignancy
    D. Usually undergoes spontaneous involution.

75. Regarding Actinic keratosis, which is false:
    A. Requires biopsy or excision for cyto-pathologic study
    B. Develops into squamous cell carcinoma in about 20% of lesions
    C. Exhibits hyperkeratosis, dyskeratosis and parakeratosis
    D. Commonly affects the eyelids.

76. Regarding capillary hemangiomas, which is false:
    A. Are usually present at birth
    B. Regress by age 7 years in 75% of affected individuals
    C. May be associated with the Kasabach-Merritt syndrome
    D. Affect girls more frequently than boys.

77. Regarding congenital melanocytic nevi, which is false:
    A. Occur in 1% of newborns
    B. May be seen in "kissing nevi" of the lids
    C. Are usually junctional nevi
    D. May degenerate into malignant melanoma.

78. Regarding the nevus of Ota, which is false:
    A. Is composed of pigmented dendritic melanocytes
    B. Is usually unilateral and congenital
    C. Often undergoes malignant degeneration in blacks
    D. Arises from dermal melanocytes.

79. Regarding molluscum contagiosum, which is false:
    A. Usually results from sexual contact and transmission in adults
    B. May produce a follicular conjunctival reaction
    C. May be confluent in immunocompromised patients
    D. Is caused by a large RNA poxvirus.

80. Regarding basal cell carcinoma, which is false:
    A. Commonly metastasizes
    B. May be pigmented
    C. Affects the lower lids in two-thirds of patients
    D. Is related to ultraviolet light exposure in fair-skinned individuals.

81. Acceptable treatment techniques for basal cell carcinoma include all except:
    A. Cryotherapy
    B. Mohs' micrographic surgery
    C. Initial radiation therapy
    D. Radiation therapy to advanced or recurrent lesions.

82. Regarding sebaceous gland carcinoma of the eyelids, which is false:
    A. Is the third most common eyelid malignancy
    B. Is more common in women than in men
    C. Must be confirmed by full thickness wedge biopsy
    D. Arises from the meibomian and moll glands.

83. Regarding malignant melanoma of eyelid skin, which is false:
    A. Is usually nodular
    B. May arise from congenital nevi
    C. May arise from acquired melanosis
    D. May be successfully treated with cryotherapy.

84. Regarding dog bites, which is false:
    A. Involve the orbit in 5 to 10% of patients especially kids

B. Contain *Pasteurella multocida* organisms in up to 50% of cases
C. Should not be primarily closed for 24 h because of rabies risk
D. From healthy dogs may contain *Capnocytophaga canimorsus* organisms, which can cause meningitis.

85. Lipogranulomatous inflammation is seen in:
    A. Fungal infection
    B. Tuberculosis
    C. Chalazion
    D. Viral infection.

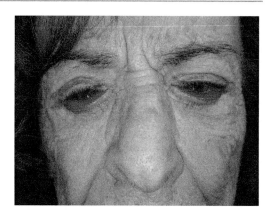

87. Regarding the above lesion:
    A. Is a stationary disease
    B. Results from laxity of the canthal tendons
    C. Treated by disinsertion of the lid retractors
    D. Can occur in both upper and lower lids.

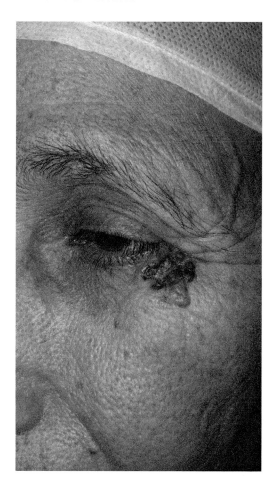

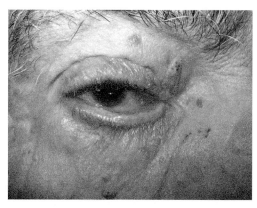

88. Regarding the above lesion, all are true except:
    A. Is caused by medial canthal laxity
    B. The lateral distraction test is positive
    C. Punctal dilatation is required in the management
    D. A medial spindle procedure is usually sufficient.

86. This raised skin lesion is likely to be which of the following?
    A. Keratoacanthoma
    B. Squamous cell carcinoma
    C. Basal cell carcinoma
    D. Malignant melanoma.

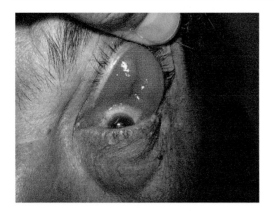

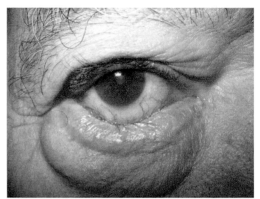

89. The above patient has chronic conjunctivitis with upper eyelids that easily evert. What additional feature of this disorder would you expect to be present?
    A. Tarsal biopsy showing decreased fibrillin
    B. History of hypoglycemia
    C. Follicular conjunctivitis
    D. History of sleep apnea.

91. Treatment of the above lesion would be best accomplished by:
    A. Suturing the orbicularis to the inferior fornix
    B. Suturing the retractors to the tarsus
    C. Suturing the orbital septum to the capsulopalpebral head
    D. Suturing the Lockwood ligament to the conjunctiva and suspensory ligament of the fornix.

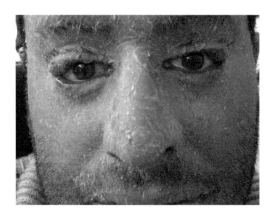

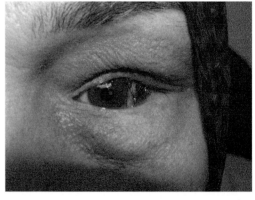

90. The above patient has:
    A. Xeroderma
    B. Icthyosis
    C. Rosacea
    D. Tuberous sclerosis.

92. What is the pathogenesis of the above lesion?:
    A. Horizontal lid laxity and eyelid retractor disinsertion
    B. Lower lid retractor dysgenesis
    C. Over-riding of preseptal orbicularis oculi muscle
    D. Vertical contracture of tarsoconjunctiva.

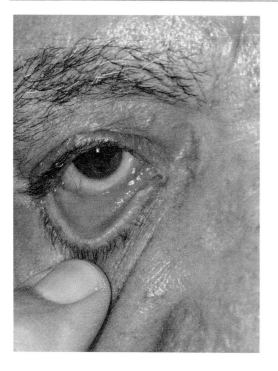

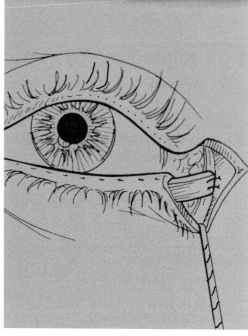

93. The above is a test of:
    A. Lateral canthal tendon weakness
    B. Medial canthal tendon weakness
    C. Tarsal weakness
    D. Orbicularis weakness.

95. The above procedure is used in the surgical
    treatment of all except:
    A. Ectropion
    B. Entropion
    C. Ptosis
    D. Lid retraction.

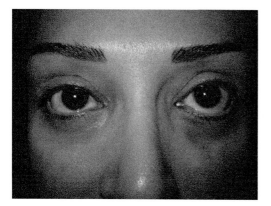

94. The most likely cause of the lesion in the
    left side is:
    A. Paralytic
    B. Mechanical
    C. Involutional
    D. Iatrogenic.

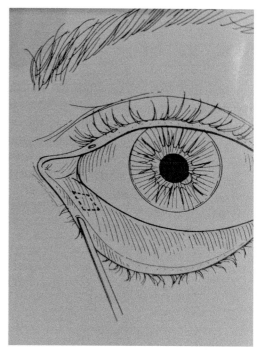

96. The mechanism by which this procedure works is:
    A. Inward shortening of the conjunctiva
    B. Dilatation and repositioning of the punctum
    C. Reinsertion of the lower lid retraction onto the tarsus
    D. Rotation of the lid margin.

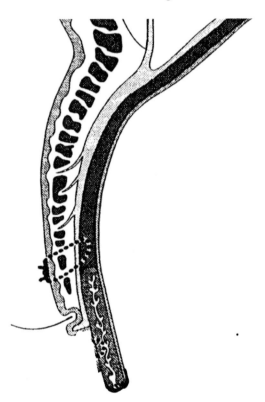

97. The above procedure is used in the treatment of:
    A. Involutional ectropion
    B. Cicatricial ectropion
    C. Involutional entropion
    D. Cicatricial entropion.

98. In a tarsal strip lateral canthoplasty, the strip is sutured to the:
    A. Opposite eyelid margin tarsus
    B. Opposite limb of the lateral canthal ligament
    C. Periosteum inside the lateral orbital rim
    D. Periosteum external to the lateral orbital rim.

99. Regarding gold weight implants, one is false:
    A. The most common procedure used for treatment of paralytic lagophthalmus
    B. The appropriate weight selection is carried out through a process of intraoperative tapping
    C. The gold weight implant is sutured to the anterior surfaces of the tarsal plate
    D. Platinum can be used as alternative.

100. In involutional ectropion, the most appropriate statement is:
    A. Caused by Skin laxity
    B. There is chronic conjunctival inflammation
    C. Presence of horizontal laxity in tarsal plate
    D. Presence of trichiasis.

101. Epicanthus inversus occurs when:
    A. Fold of skin is most prominent in the upper eyelid
    B. Fold of skin is most prominent in the lower eyelid
    C. Fold of skin is distributed equally in the upper and lower lids
    D. Fold of skin arises from the caruncle.

102. In the surgical treatment of upper lid retraction due to thyroid associated ophthalmopathy, which is correct:
    A. Contraindicated in exposure keratopathy
    B. Can be corrected with excision of Müller muscle
    C. Insertion of a spacer between the Müller muscle and levator aponeurosis
    D. Lateral tarsorrhapy is the surgical modality of choice.

103. Quickert sutures:
    A. Have a long lasting effect
    B. Are used for ectropion
    C. Involve lateral tarsal strip
    D. Are used for reinsertion of the retractors.

104. Regarding entropion the least appropriate statement is:
    A. Acute spastic entropion follows sclera buckle procedure
    B. Involutional entropion is usually associated with the lower lid
    C. An inferior fornix that is deeper than normal may indicate lower lid retractors disinsertion
    D. The lateral tarsal strip operation is useful.

105. Which one of the following would be the best treatment for a patient with typical Bell's palsy with severe corneal exposure?
    A. Temporary lateral tarsorrhaphy
    B. Pentagonal wedge resection of the lower eyelid
    C. Punctual electrocautery
    D. Inferior retractor recession with full-thickness skin grafting of the lower lid.

106. Etiological factors in involutional entropion,one is false:
    A. Horizontal eyelid laxity
    B. Shortening of the anterior lamella
    C. Laxity of eyelid retractors
    D. Overriding presptal orbicularis muscle.

107. The surgical procedures to correct lid retraction with lateral flare include all except:
    A. Recession of the levator aponrurosis with space
    B. Measured myotomy of the levator muscle with lateral tarsorrhaphy
    C. Full thickness transverse blepharotomy
    D. Lid splitting, lateral tarsorrhaphy with recession of lid retractors.

108. Clinical clues to the disinsertion of the lower lid retractors include all of the following EXCEPT:
    A. White line below the tarsal border caused by the dehisced edge of the disinserted retactors
    B. Higher than normal lower eyelid position
    C. Decreased movement of the lower lid on downgaze
    D. Shrinking of the inferior conjunctival fornix.

109. Which one of the following is the LEAST common form of ectropion?
    A. Congenital
    B. Paralytic
    C. Mechanical
    D. Cicatricial.

110. Repair of lower eyelid involutional entropion would be BEST accomplished by:
    A. Suturing the orbicularis to the inferior fornix
    B. Suturing the retractors to the tarsus
    C. Suturing the orbital septum to the capsulopalpebral head
    D. Suturing the Lockwood's ligament to the conjunctiva and suspensory ligament of the fornix.

111. The most common cause of upper eyelid retraction is:
    A. Recession of the superior rectus muscle
    B. Congenital eyelid retraction
    C. Surgical overcorrection of blepharoptosis
    D. Thyroid eye disease.

112. The following are true about the facial nerve EXCEPT:
    A. Does not contain sensory nerves
    B. Supplies secretomotor fibers to the submandibular glands
    C. Exits the skull through the styloid foramen
    D. Lies lateral to the external carotid artery within the parotid gland.

113. What is the pathogenesis of acute spastic entropion?
    A. Horizontal lid laxity and eyelid retractor disinsertion
    B. Ocular irritation or inflammation
    C. Over-riding of preseptal orbicularis oculi muscle
    D. Vertical contracture of tarsoconjunctiva.

114. A 65 year old male develops inturning of both lower lid margins. Ophthalmic examination reveals a white subconjunctival line several millimetres below the inferior

tarsal border with no movement of the lower lid on downgaze. What pathology has happened in these lower eyelids?
A. Cicatrization of the tarsoconjunctiva
B. Disinsertion of the lower lid retractors
C. Horizontal lower lid laxity
D. Symblepharon.

115. Cicatricial entropion is generally associated with all except:
A. Trichiasis
B. Anterior lamellar shortage
C. Blepharospasm
D. Symblepharon.

116. A 50 year old female presents with inward turning of both lower lid margins. Ophthalmic examination reveals chronic conjunctival inflammation in both eyes with the diagnosis of ocular cicatricial pemphigoid. What is the appropriate plan of action?
A. Anti-inflammatory therapy and surgery for entropion
B. Corneal shielding and anti-inflammatory therapy only
C. Corneal shielding and anti-inflammatory therapy then surgery for entropion
D. Corneal shielding and surgery for entropion then anti-inflammatory therapy.

117. A 50 year old male presents with outward turning of the left lower eyelid margin. The patient has no other significant history. Ophthalmic examination reveals a large chalazion in the left lower eyelid. What treatment is indicated for correction of the lower eyelid margin malposition?
A. Chalazion incision and curettage
B. Lateral and medial canthal tightening
C. Lateral tarsal strip procedure
D. Medial spindle procedure.

118. When is Van Millingen's operation indicated?
A. Trichiasis & entropion of upper eyelid
B. Pure trichiasis of upper eyelid
C. Trichiasis & entropion of lower eyelid
D. Pure trichiasis of lower eyelid.

119. The operation of plication of inferior lid retractors is indicated in:
A. Senile ectropion
B. Senile entropion
C. Cicatricial entropion
D. Paralytic ectropion.

120. Fibrous attachment of the lid to the eyeball is called:
A. Symblepharon
B. Entropion
C. Ectropion
D. Ankyloblepharon.

121. Telecanthus means:
A. Widened interpupillary distance
B. Widened root of nose with normal interpupillary distance
C. Widely separated medial orbital wall
D. Widely separated canthi.

122. Distichiasis means:
A. Increased number of eyelashes in the lower lid
B. Second row of eyelashes
C. Increased thickness of eyelashes
D. Increased pigmentation of eyelashes.

123. In facial nerve palsy; Prevention of gold weight exposure is best achieved by:
A. Using a small gold weight implant
B. Using a large gold weight implant
C. Inserting the weight under the orbicularis muscle
D. Meticulous suture closure of the skin.

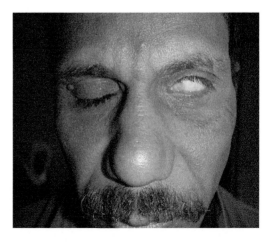

124. Surgical management of the shown patient includes all of the following, except
    A. Gold weight implantation
    B. Lower lid tightening procedure
    C. Blepharoplasty
    D. Brow lifting.

125. All of the following may occur in a patient with a palsy of the seventh cranial nerve, except
    A. Epiphora
    B. Keratitis
    C. Ectropion
    D. Ptosis.

126. All of the following are characteristic of blepharophimosis except
    A. Autosomal dominant
    B. Lower eyelid entropion
    C. Deformed ears
    D. Hypoplasia of the superior orbital rims.

127. A patient undergoes placement of hard palate graft for lower eyelid retraction. Which of the following best characterizes the epithelium of the graft?
    A. Retention of native epithelium
    B. Metaplasia into nonkeratinized epithelium
    C. Survival of submucosal glands
    D. Conjunctivalization of epithelium.

128. An old patient has chronic left eye irritation. He has a snap back test of greater than 6 mm and normal palpebral and forniceal conjunctiva. all of the following are true, except:
    A. No inferior movement of lower eyelid during down gaze
    B. Deeper than usual inferior fornix
    C. Presence of a white subconjunctival line below the inferior tarsal border
    D. Lower than normal position of lower eyelid.

129. Which statement about eyelid abnormalities is false?
    A. Congenital coloboma of the eyelid always involves the lower eyelid and can vary from a small notch to a complete absence of the eyelid

    B. Cryptophthalmos is a rare condition that is caused by a lack of differentiation of eyelid structures and is characterized by absence of a palpebral fissure with uninterrupted skin from the forehead over the eye to the skin of the cheek
    C. Ankyloblepharon filiforme adnatum is a form of ankyloblepharon in which the eyelid margins are connected by thin strands of tissue
    D. Distichiasis is a condition in which an accessory row of eyelashes grows from or are posterior to the meibomian orifices.

130. Trachoma can cause all of the following changes *except*:
    A. Distichiasis
    B. Punctal stenosis
    C. Conjunctival scarring
    D. Entropion.

131. All of the following pairs match mechanisms of involutional entropion with the surgical repair except:
    A. Horizontal lower lid laxity-lateral tarsal strip
    B. Dehiscence of the lower lid retractors-retractor advancement
    C. Overriding of the pretarsal orbicularis by the preseptal orbicularis-excision of a strip of preseptal orbicularis
    D. Inward rotation of the lid by steatoblepharon-lower lid blepharoplasty.

132. An old patient with a previous stroke lives in a nursing home. He is on oral anticoagulants.The patient continually complains of foreign-body sensation and discharge n one eye. Which of the following procedures is most appropriate In this setting?
    A. Rattachment of the capsulopalpebral fascia
    B. A lateral tarsal strip procedure
    C. Rotational sutures (Quickert sutures)
    D. Tarsal wedge excision.

133. Which one of the following is likely to occur, with respect to the epithelium, of the transplanted tissue of a hard palate graft?
 A. It will maintain some form of keratinization (orthokeratosis and/or parakeratosis)
 B. It will remain fully keratinized
 C. It will convert from keratinized to nonkeratinized
 D. All epithelium will be lost.

134. How does lower eyelid retractor repair for involutional entropion of the lower eyelid work by?
 A. Reattaching the capsulopalpebral fascia to the tarsus
 B. Shortening the septum
 C. Repairing cicatricial changes
 D. Horizontally shortening the orbicularis.

135. What is the most common complaint following successful correction of paralytic ectropion?
 A. Consecutive entropion
 B. Prolonged chemosis
 C. Persistent epiphora
 D. Overelevation of the lateral canthal angle.

136. When performing a lateral tarsal strip for horizontal lid laxity of the lower lid, what is the correct placement of the lateral canthus?
 A. 2 mm lower than the medial canthus
 B. 2 mm above the medial canthus
 C. Outside the lateral orbital rim
 D. At Lockwood's tubercle.

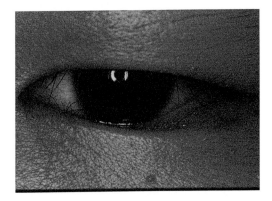

137. What is the pathophysiologic mechanism underlying this condition?
 A. Laxity of the tarsal plat
 B. Abnormal attachment of the orbital septum
 C. Abnormal attachment of the skin and orbicularis oculi muscle
 D. Laxity of the canthal tendons.

138. Ectropion and loss of eyelashes should alert one to the possibility of which one of the following?
 A. Facial nerve (VII) palsy
 B. Chronic eyelid webbing
 C. Involutional ectropion
 D. Malignancy.

139. Unilateral rounding of the medial canthal tendon is a feature of which disorder?
 A. Fracture of the medial wall of the orbit
 B. Connective tissue disease involving the medial canthal tendon
 C. Lacrimal sac tumor
 D. Avulsion of the medial canthal tendon.

140. A Quickert suture is most effectively used when repairing what disorder?
 A. Spastic entropion
 B. Distichiasis
 C. Involutional entropion
 D. Cicatricial entropion.

141. A 4-year-old child is referred for bilateral epiphora. Examination shows eyelashes on both lower eyelids rubbing against the inferior cornea. The parents state that an older sibling has the similar symptoms, which resolved without treatment. What is the most likely diagnosis?
 A. Entropion
 B. Epiblepharon
 C. Euryblepharon
 D. Trichiasis.

142. What is the preferred treatment for cicatricial ectropion?
 A. Lateral tarsal strip plus repair of lower eyelid retractors

B. Lateral tarsal strip plus skin graft

C. Fascia lata suspension of the lower eyelid

D. Lateral tarsal strip plus medial spindle procedure.

143. What term describes an abnormally wide distance between the medial canthi in the presence of a normal interpupillary distance?
    A. Exorbitism
    B. Hypertelorism
    C. Telorbitism
    D. Telecanthus.

144. Which is incorrect; Eyelid retraction may:
    A. Result from Muller's muscle stimulation alone
    B. Be declared when the lower lid margin is below the limbus
    C. Be caused by seventh nerve palsy
    D. Be a manifestation of Hering's law in the setting of contralateral ptosis.

145. Neurogenic causes of eyelid retraction does not include:
    A. Dorsal midbrain syndrome
    B. Wernicke's encephalopathy
    C. Palatal myoclonus
    D. Impending tentorial herniation.

146. Myogenic causes of eyelid retraction does not include:
    A. Myasthenia gravis
    B. Graves' dysthyroid orbitopathy
    C. Familial periodic paralysis
    D. Down syndrome.

147. Regarding entropion, which is incorrect:
    A. Is often caused by attenuation of the capsulopalpebral fascia and orbital septum
    B. May be caused by age-related horizontal lower lid laxity
    C. Is commonly caused by enophthalmos
    D. May be caused by reduced posterior lid lamellar support.

148. Entropion may be mimicked by all except:
    A. Epiblepharon
    B. Distichiasis
    C. Trichiasis
    D. Symblepharon.

149. Regarding techniques for entropion repair, which is incorrect:
    A. Lid retractor reattachment
    B. Botulinum toxin injection
    C. Transverse tarsorrhaphy
    D. Kuhnt-Szymanowski procedure.

150. Ectropion has been associated with all except:
    A. Medial or lateral canthal tendon laxity
    B. Orbicularis muscle weakness
    C. Cicatricial skin changes
    D. Tightening of the inferior lid retractors.

151. Techniques available for correction of ectropion include all except:
    A. Lateral tarsal strip procedure
    B. Full-thickness wedge excision
    C. Y-plasty
    D. Medial canthal tendon resection.

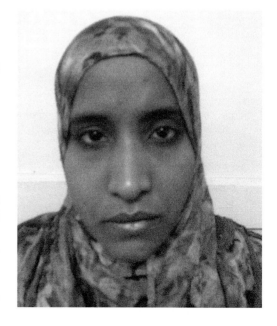

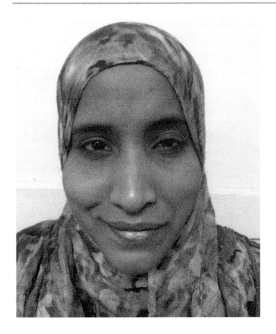

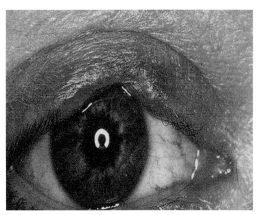

154. The above photo is a reported complication of:
    A. Electrolysis
    B. Diathery
    C. Cryotherapy
    D. Laser therapy.

152. The above patient has:
    A. Jaw winking syndrome
    B. Aberrant regeneration of 3rd nerve
    C. Aberrant regeneration of 7th nerve
    D. Duane syndrome.

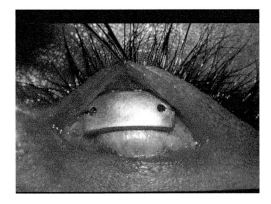

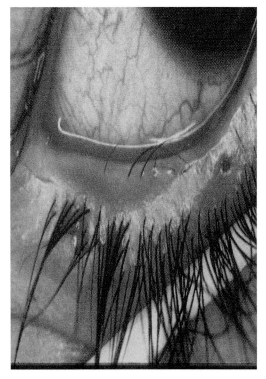

153. The surgical technique shown in the figure includes all except:
    A. Intraoperative choice of the proper implant
    B. Fixation to tarsus with nylon sutures
    C. Closure in two layers
    D. Recession of the levator muscle.

155. The above figure is an example of:
    A. Trichiasis
    B. Distichiasis
    C. Entropion
    D. Epibleharon.

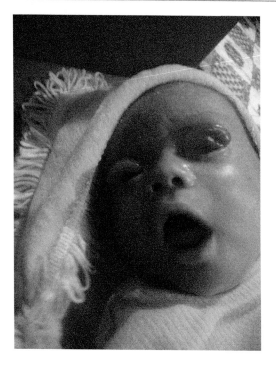

156. The above anomaly is best treated by:
   A. Intense lubrication
   B. Immediate reduction and tarsorraphy
   C. Cinjunctival excision
   D. Horizontal lid shortening.

157. Blepharitis is:
   A. An acute inflammation of the lid margin
   B. A chronic inflammation of the lid margin
   C. Inflammation of the eyelid skin
   D. Inflammation of the eyelid skin and underlying soft tissues.

158. What is the most effective treatment of active trachoma?
   A. Single dose of 1gm oral azithromycin
   B. Topical neomycin ointment
   C. Topical fucidic acid ointment
   D. Topical quinolone drops.

159. Which of the followings statements about conjunctival biopsy in Ocular Cicatricial Pemphigoid (OCP) is true:
   A. The part of specimen for immunofluorescence analysis should be submitted in formalin

B. Immunofluorescence demonstrates IgG, IgM positivity in the epithelial basement membrane zone
   C. A negative result of immunofluorescence rule out possibility of OCP
   D. Histology shows subepithelial band of inflammatory cells, predominantly neutrophils.

160. Regarding tarsal rotation procedures, all are correct except:
   A. Can be done transcutaneously
   B. Can be done transconjunctivally
   C. Requires a tarsus that is not deformed or atrophic
   D. Requires more than 3 sutures to induce rotation.

161. The centurion syndrome is characterized by:
   A. Epiphora in young adults
   B. Low Hertel exophthalmometer readings
   C. Patent nasolacrimal system on irrigation
   D. Favorable response to intubation.

162. The management of the centurion syndrome may include all except:
   A. Disinsertion of both limbs of the medial canthal tendon
   B. Disinsertion of only the anterior limb of the medial canthal tendon
   C. Medial spindle procedure
   D. Lower eyelid retractor plication.

163. Regarding floppy eyelid syndrome, the most appropriate statement is:
   A. Presence of follicular conjunctivitis
   B. Obesity is a strong association
   C. Sleeping supine is a risk factor
   D. No surgical management is required condition usually resolves with conservative management.

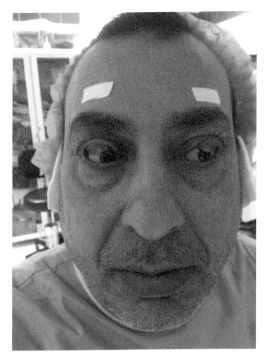

164. Which of the following is characteristic of the histopathology of the above condition?
  A. Decrease in tarsal elastin fibers
  B. Decrease in conjunctival elastin fibres
  C. Decrease in tarsal collagen type I
  D. Decrease in tarsal collagen type III.

165. A mildly obese patient complains of chronic irritation in both eyes which is worse in the morning. In one eye, the patient has ptosis. What question would address a risk factor for the patient's ptosis?
  A. Do you sleep face down?
  B. Do you suffer from recurring, unilateral facial spasms?
  C. Do you suffer from dementia?
  D. Do you have a history of Bell's palsy?

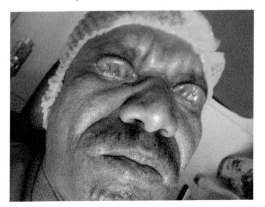

166. Patients with the above condition has blepharoptosis in one or both eyes. Which of the following statements accurately describes the surgical approach to their form of ptosis?
  A. Frontalis suspension is often required to provide adequate eyelid elevation and contour
  B. Levator advancement/resection is not useful when treating this disorder
  C. Horizontal shortening of the upper lid is often enough to elevate the affected lid
  D. Lash ptosis does not respond to horizontal tightening of the eyelid.

167. A patient presents with obesity, a soft rubbery tarsus, watery tearing, and mucus discharge from one eye. He prefers to sleep in a face down position. What surgical treatment would be preferred to improve his symptom?
  A. Horizontal eyelid tightening
  B. Canthotomy of lateral canthal tendon
  C. Canthotomy of superior limb of lateral canthus
  D. Vertical shortening of tarsus.

168. The S in the SAFE strategy can be all except:
  A. Bilamellar tarsal rotation procedure
  B. Transconjunctival tarsal rotation procedure
  C. Lateral tarsal strip procedure
  D. Surgical resection of maldirected lashes.

169. Regarding trachoma staging, TF means:
  A. Trachomatous inflammation-follicular
  B. Trachomatous inflammation–intense
  C. Trachomatous conjuctival scarring
  D. Trachomatous trichiasis.

170. Regarding trachoma staging, TI means:
  A. Trachomatous inflammation-follicular
  B. Trachomatous inflammation–intense
  C. Trachomatous conjuctival scarring
  D. Trachomatous trichiasis.

171. Regarding trachoma staging, the blinding stage is:
    A. TF
    B. TS
    C. TI
    D. CO.

172. Upper motor neuron facial nerve lesion results in:
    A. Bilateral paralysis of the upper facial muscles
    B. Bilateral paralysis of the lower facial muscles

C. Ipsilateral paralysis of the lower facial muscles
D. Contralateral paralysis of the lower facial muscles.

173. A 52-year-old male patient has a growing eyelid lesion. He has a strong family history for colonic cancer. Ophthalmic examination reveals lid changes suggestive of sebaceous cell carcinoma. What is the most likely diagnosis?
    A. Bazex syndrome
    B. Gardner syndrome
    C. Gorlin-Golz syndrome
    D. Muir-Torre syndrome.

Answers in this chapter lid lesions

1	A	22	B	43	A	64	B	85	C	106	B	127	A			168	C
2	A	23	B	44	D	65	B	86	D	107	D	128	D	148	D	169	A
3	A	24	D	45	B	66	C	87	B	108	D	129	A	149	D	170	B
4	C	25	D	46	A	67	B	88	C	109	A	130	A	150	D	171	D
5	C	26	A	47	B	68	A	89	D	110	B	131	D	151	C	172	D
6	D	27	A	48	D	69	B	90	B	111	D	132	C	152	C	173	D
7	D	28	B	49	B	70	D	91	B	112	A	133	A	153	A		
8	B	29	A	50	A	71	D	92	D	113	B	134	A	154	C		
9	A	30	A	51	C	72	C	93	D	114	B	135	C	155	D		
10	C	31	D	52	D	73	C	94	D	115	B	136	B	156	B		
11	B	32	C	53	D	74	B	95	C	116	C	137	C	157	B		
12	A	33	C	54	C	75	D	96	C	117	A	138	D	158	A		
13	B	34	C	55	C	76	A	97	D	118	B	139	D	159	B		
14	C	35	C	56	C	77	C	98	C	119	B	140	C	160	D		
15	D	36	C	57	B	78	C	99	B	120	A	141	B	161	D		
16	C	37	B	58	C	79	D	100	B	121	B	142	B	162	A		
17	C	38	A	59	A	80	A	101	B	122	B	143	D	163	B		
18	A	39	A	60	D	81	C	102	B	123	C	144	B	164	A		
19	B	40	B	61	A	82	D	103	D	124	C	145	B	165	A		
20	C	41	B	62	D	83	D	104	A	125	D	146	D	166	C		
21	B	42	B	63	A	84	C	105	A	126	B	147	C	167	A		

Ptosis

3

Essam A. El Toukhy

Blepharoptosis refers to drooping of the upper eyelid and is one of the most common surgical eyelid disorders. It can occur in both children and adults, and can be classified based on the aetiology of the ptosis: neurogenic, myogenic, aponeurotic, mechanical and pseudoptosis.

Ptosis is the most common lid malposition encountered in clinical practice in both adults and children population and is the most surgically correctable lid disorder.

The upper lid position is a function of the delicate balance between the lid retractors including levator muscle, Muller's muscle, and frontalis muscle, and the lid protractors including the orbital pat and palpebral part of the orbicularis oculi muscle.

Normally the upper lid covers the upper 1–2 mm of the cornea in the primary position, providing no obstacle to image formation on the retina. It follows the globe on looking down with no lag. It provides complete coverage of the eye on lid closure. Finally, it rises up for up to 20 mm in extreme up-gaze.

Changing the activity of the levator and Muller's muscles, brings all of these movements about. The frontalis muscles are called into action only in extreme up-gaze. The orbicularis muscle in mainly used in forceful lid closure

although its palpebral part shares in the blinking mechanisms.

Both upper eyelids are symmetrical. The brain considers both lid retractor as yoke muscle. They receive equal innervations form single subdivision of the oculomotor nucleus in the midbrain. Changes in the position of one lid will lead to affection of the position of the other.

Evaluation of the ptotic patient should include an attempt to determine the precise aetiology of the ptosis. Congenital ptosis is a localized dystrophy of the levator muscle. There is fibrous tissue where striated muscle would be expected. This correlates well with the severity of the ptosis. Mueller's muscle is normal. Congenital ptosis may be unilateral or bilateral. It maybe classified as simple or complicated by ophthalmoplegia (superior rectus weakness), blepharophimosis syndrome, and Marcus Gunn jawing winking ptosis.

Patients may have amblyopia resulting from anisometropia, strabismus, pupil occlusion, or meridional amblyopia.

In congenital ptosis; the indication for doing ptosis surgery is a child who has an eyelid obstructing the visual axis, amblyopia, abnormal head position or unsatisfactory facial appearance. The best time for surgery is around 4 years of age when accurate measurements can be taken unless the risk of amblyopia and poor visual development is high. Most cases of ptosis correction are done under general anesthesia.

E. A. El Toukhy (✉)
Oculoplasty Service, Cairo University, Cairo, Egypt
e-mail: eeltoukhy@yahoo.com

© The Author(s), under exclusive license to Springer Nature Switzerland AG 2021
E. A. El Toukhy (ed.), *Oculoplasty for Ophthalmologists*, https://doi.org/10.1007/978-3-030-68469-3_3

37

However older children around 16–17 years of age may be performed under monitored anesthesia to allow for the best eyelid height and contour.

In adults, the most common cause of ptosis is aponeurotic (also known as senile ptosis). In this condition, the levator muscle is normal, but the levator aponeurosis is either attenuated or has undergone dehiscence from its normal insertions on the tarsal plate and in the orbicularis muscle. This may be a naturally occurring involutional change, or it may be precipitated by intraocular surgery, long-term daily contact lens wear, steroid use or trauma.

Ptosis surgery for adults is one of the most commonly performed procedures by Oculoplastic surgeons. A detailed preoperative history and clinical evaluation are crucial for determining the cause of ptosis and the best procedure for the individual patient. Many surgical procedures have been described to correct ptosis, each with its own indications and advantages. The individual success of any of these procedures depends on its ability to adjust the eyelid position relative to the amount of levator function present. Ptosis surgery can be broadly classified according to whether it is targeting the posterior upper lid retractor (Müller's muscle), anterior upper lid retractor (levator aponeurosis) or the brow (frontalis muscle). Each procedure has its distinct advantages and own set of complications. A thorough knowledge of the steps and nuances of each procedure will enable the surgeon to better use them for the right patients and optimize surgical outcomes.

Levator advancement or resection surgery remains the standard of adult ptosis surgery especially in patients with moderate to severe ptosis with fair to normal levator function, who require simultaneous blepharoplasty, do not respond to phenylephrine or want lid crease formation. Although most appropriate for acquired aponeurotic ptosis, this surgery also works well for neurogenic, myogenic and congenital ptosis. It allows for accurate adjustment of eyelid height and contour, especially when performed under local anaesthesia. In most cases with fair to good levator muscle function,

levator advancement or repair is a good option for correction of ptosis, with reported success rates of 70% to more than 95%. Compared to MMCR and Fasanella-Servat, it has a clear pathophysiologic-anatomical basis of repair: reapproximation of the attenuated/dehisced levator aponeurosis back to its former anatomical position.

The "Age of aponeurotic awareness" directed the trend of ptosis surgery toward the anterior approach. The proponents of levator aponeurosis surgery argued that since the defect of involutional ptosis was found to be in the aponeurosis instead of in the Müller's muscle or tarsus, it was improper to violate tissues not directly responsible for the disease as per posterior approach ptosis surgery.

Müller's muscle-conjunctival resection (MMCR), or conjunctivomüllerectomy, is a good option for correction of mild to moderate upper eyelid ptosis with good levator muscle function and positive response to phenylephrine preoperatively. Unlike the Fasanella-Servat procedure, MMCR preserves the tarsus and accessory glands and has several advantages: predictable, relatively simple to perform, lack of an external scar, and ability to maintain a natural upper eyelid contour

In patients with no or very poor levator function, the operation that will achieve adequate eyelid elevation is frontalis suspension. In adult ptosis surgery, this is reserved for patients with pre-existing congenital ptosis, myogenic or neurogenic ptosis which cannot be corrected with conventional ptosis surgery on the levator muscle. In this procedure, the frontalis is used as a supplemental eyelid retractor as the eyelid is fixed to the frontalis muscle at the brow. The patient opens the eye by elevating the brow and closes the eye by contracting the orbicularis.

Frontalis suspension surgery may use several surgical techniques and different sling materials. Materials include autogenous or banked fascia lata and alloplastic materials that include chromic gut, collagen, polypropylene, silicone, stainless steel, silk, nylon monofilament, polyester and polytetrafluoroethylene (PTFE). Autogenous fascia lata has proven to give good results with comparably low rates of recurrent ptosis and infections but requires secondary surgery on the leg for harvesting of the fascia.

The frontalis muscle flap advancement is a technique of direct transfer of the force of the frontalis muscle to the eyelid without the insertion of fascia, suture or a graft between the muscle and the tarsus. Frontalis suspension by frontalis muscle flap is a well-accepted method of treating severe bleharoptosis. Being from the same patient, there is no risk of rejection or severe body reaction as may occur with homogenous or alloplastic materials. There is no risk of disease transmission. A Frontalis flap grows with the child's growth and does not lead to cheese-wiring as synthetic materials. The frontalis muscle is well developed before fascia lata maturation. Therefore, this procedure can be performed earlier, if indicated, in cases of congenital ptosis. Additional advantages of this technique include its technical simplicity, lack of remote scar as the donor site is in the primary surgical field, minimal ptosis on upgaze, less lid lag on downgaze, preservation of eyelid contour and less tendency for the lid to pull away from the eye. In contrast to traditional frontalis slings, only one 2 cm brow incision is required. This direct linkage of the frontalis muscle to the eyelid has been documented by postoperative magnetic resonance imaging scan.

Blepharoptosis will continue to be a commonly presented condition to the ophthalmologist and oculoplastic surgeon, given its interference with the patients' visual field and quality of life. Numerous surgical techniques have been described in the management of blepharoptosis. The choice of treatment is dependent upon the severity of the patient's ptosis, the levator function, the response to phenylephrine, and the surgeon's preference. Levator advancement or resection surgery remains the standard of adult ptosis surgery especially in patients with moderate to severe

ptosis with fair to normal levator function, who require simultaneous blepharoplasty, do not respond to phenylephrine or want lid crease formation. Patients who demonstrate mild-to-moderate ptosis (<3 mm) with sufficient levator function (>8 mm) may benefit from the posterior lamellar approach, mainly involving Müller's muscle-conjunctival resection (MMCR) with or without tarsectomy. The frontalis suspension is less frequently used in adult ptosis surgery but is useful in cases with very poor or absent levator function such as pre-existing congenital ptosis, neurogenic or myogenic ptosis.

Marcus-Gunn ptosis and the blepharophimosis syndrome are special types of ptosis that deserves special mention.

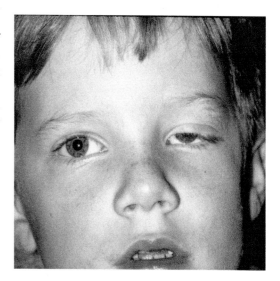

Ptosis

1. A patient present with unilateral ptosis associated with poor levator function, the most appropriate surgical procedure is:
   A. Unilateral frontalis suspension
   B. Maximal external levator resection
   C. Fasanella-Servat
   D. Mullerectomy.

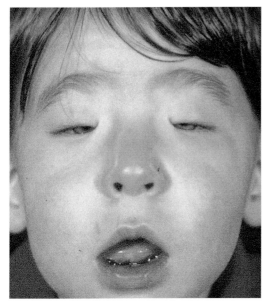

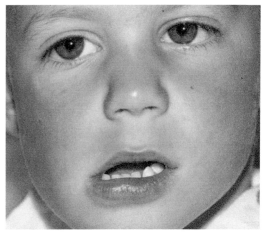

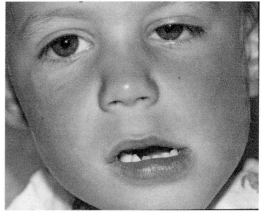

2. The following is a feature of the above disorder:
    A. Autosomal Recessive
    B. Reduced intercanthal distance
    C. Epicanthus inversus
    D. Horizontal lid deficiency.

3. Blepharophimosis syndrome, one is false:
    A. It is an autosomal recessive
    B. Usually present with telecanthus
    C. Lower eyelid ectropion
    D. Hypoplasia of the superior orbital rim.

4. Blepharophimosis is generally associated with, one is false:
    A. Ptosis
    B. Epicanthus inversus
    C. Distichiasis
    D. Ectropion.

5. Neurogenic ptosis is:
    A. Associated with congenital cranial nerve VI palsy
    B. Associated with congenital Horner syndrome
    C. Associated with abduction defect in eye movement
    D. Frontalis suspension is contraindicated due to risk of lagophthalmous.

6. The above is:
    A. Is a form of acquired synkinetic neurogenic ptosis
    B. Caused by aberrant connections between CN V and levator muscle
    C. Vasculopathic or compressive lesion must be excluded
    D. Pupil is usually involved.

7. Regarding acquired myogenic ptosis, the least appropriate statement is:
    A. Associated with muscular dystrophy
    B. Surgical procedure is directed towards levator muscle
    C. Frontalis suspension is used for treatment
    D. Secondary exposure keratitis can result after surgical correction.

8. Fasanella-Servat operation is useful in which specific case of ptosis?
   A. Minimal ptosis
   B. Ptosis with myasthenia
   C. Horner's syndrome
   D. Congenital ptosis.

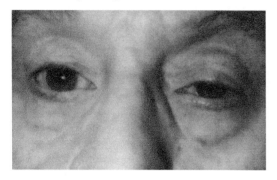

9. A 70-year-old woman presents to you with a 3 mm left upper eyelid ptosis with a high eyelid crease and normal levator function. The appropriate treatment of choice is?
   A. Posterior approach standard mullerectomy
   B. Levator aponeurosis advancement
   C. Internal tarsoconjunctival resection (Fasanella-Servat operation)
   D. Frontalis muscle suspension using a silicone rod to allow postoperative adjustment.

10. A 12-year-old girl with repeated swelling and ptosis of both upper eyelids complain of repeated episodes of eyelid inflammation and swelling. What is the most likely diagnosis?
    A. Dermatochalasis
    B. Steatoblepharon
    C. Blepharospasm
    D. Blepharochalasis.

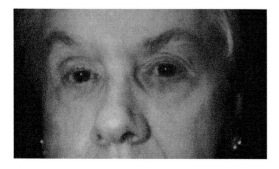

11. In this patient with ptosis post cataract surgery with good levator function and a high or effaced upper eyelid crease, what would be your procedure of choice?
    A. Levator muscle resection
    B. Reinsertion of levator aponeurosis
    C. Muller's muscle resection
    D. Bilateral frontalis suspension.

12. The most important determinant in selecting a corrective procedure for any type of ptosis is:
    A. Vertical height of the palpebral fissure
    B. Age of the patient
    C. Amount of levator function
    D. duration of ptosis.

13. All of the following consider ptosis as a functional problem that requires correction, one is false:
    A. Ptosis with significant loss of superior field
    B. Ptosis with difficulty in reading
    C. Ptosis that causes sleepy appearance
    D. Ptosis that interferes with daily activity.

14. The poor long term outcome in frontalis suspension surgery is reported with the use of:
    A. Autogenous tensor fascia lata
    B. Banked fascia lata
    C. Silicon rods
    D. Gortex suture.

15. The most common complication of ptosis surgery is:
    A. Under correction
    B. Over correction
    C. Eyelid crease asymmetry
    D. Lagophthamus with exposure.

16. Which of the following is NOT a feature of congenital myogenic ptosis?
    A. Levator muscle tissue is replaced by fibrous or adipose tissue.
    B. Prominent upper lid crease
    C. Lid lag on down gaze
    D. Lagophthalmos.

17. All of the followings can lead to neurogenic ptosis except
    A. Horner's Syndrome
    B. Deep superior sulcus
    C. Guillain–Barré syndrome
    D. Aberrant regeneration of the oculomotor nerve.

18. The procedure of choice for moderate unilateral ptosis with good levator function and a normal upper lid crease
    A. Levator muscle resection
    B. Mullerectomy
    C. Reinsertion of levator aponeurosis
    D. Whitnall sling.

19. A 70-years old female has 4 mm of right upper lid ptosis and 1 mm of left upper eye lid retraction with high eye lid crease on the right side, with normal levator function of both lids. Treatment of choice is
    A. A moderate levator recession of the left upper eye lid
    B. A levator aponeurosis advancement on the right lid
    C. A posterior approach standard mullerectomy on the right upper eye lid
    D. A frontalis muscle suspension on the right eye lid using silicone strap to allow postoperative adjustment.

20. Which statement regarding fat encountered during eyelid surgery is FALSE?
    A. Preaponeurotic fat is orbital fat
    B. Extraconal orbital fat is an important landmark in identifying the levator aponeurosis
    C. The removal of fat from the upper eyelid nasal, central and lateral fat pads may be done with impunity
    D. In the upper eyelid, the nasal fat pad is small, whereas the lateral fat pad is the small fat pad in the lower eyelid.

21. Which one of the following is found in the blepharophimosis syndrome?
    A. Euryblepharon
    B. Ankyloblepharon

C. Epiblebharon
D. Telecanthus.

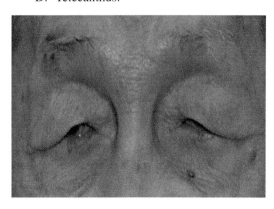

22. The proper surgical procedure for repair of this ptotic upper eyelid exhibiting a high eyelid crease, a margin to reflex distance (MRD) of 0 mm, and excellent levator function would be:
    A. Resection of the superior tarsal muscle
    B. Unilateral frontalis suspension using autogenous fascia lata
    C. Reattachment of the dehisced levator eponeurosis
    D. Plication of the levator muscle (16 mm).

23. The most common form of blepharoptosis is:
    A. Involutional blepharoptosis (aponeurotic ptosis)
    B. Neurogenic blepharoptosis
    C. Myogenic blepharoptosis
    D. Mechanical blepharoptosis.

24. In myogenic congenital ptosis, the levator complex (in the ptotic eye) is:
    A. Disinserted from the tarsus
    B. Histologically different from normal levator complex with decreased muscle fibers and fatty infiltrates
    C. Innervervated by cranial nerve VII
    D. Absent below Whitnall's ligament.

25. In patients with ptosis, the 2.5% phenylephrine hydrochloride test:
    A. Will activate the sympathetic receptors in Müller's muscle, resulting in elevation of the lid

B. Can be used to assess the approximate elevation of the lid with external levator advancement

C. Dilates the pupil so that the contralateral eyelid may drop

D. Does not affect blood pressure through systemic absorption of the phenylephrine.

26. Materials used for frontalis suspension of the eyelid include all of the following EXCEPT:
    A. Silicone
    B. Gore—Tex
    C. Supramid
    D. Polyglactin 910 (Vicryl).

27. Regarding The levator muscle, which is false:
    A. Is attached to the lesser wing of the sphenoid bone
    B. Is attached to the circle of Zinn
    C. Turns from muscle into aponeurosis where ligament of Whitnall is found
    D. Is penetrated by the superior division of the oculomotor nerve at the posterior one-third and anterior two-third junction.

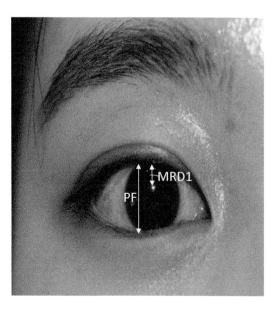

28. Which measurement represents the margin reflex distance 1 (MRD1)?
    A. Difference between vertical fissure height of both eyes
    B. From corneal light reflex to lower lid margin
    C. From corneal light reflex to upper lid margin
    D. From upper lid to lower lid margin.

29. A 70 year old female that has been diabetic for the preceding 20 years presents with right total ptosis. Ophthalmic examination is unremarkable except for right exotropia. What is the appropriate plan of management?
    A. Frontalis sling operation
    B. Frontalis sling operation with medial rectus resection
    C. Levator resection with medial rectus resection
    D. Observe for 3–6 months for spontaneous resolution.

30. What of the following is a sign of Horner's Syndrome?
    A. Head tilt
    B. Diplopia
    C. Mydriasis
    D. Mild Ptosis.

31. As regard ptosis:
    A. Levator function is good in senile ptosis
    B. Lid lag on downgaze is a feature of senile ptosis
    C. Raised skin crease is a feature of congenital ptosis
    D. The most common abnormality in congenital ptosis is in the levator appeneurosis.

32. Myasthenia patients are at higher risk for all of the following except;
    A. Thymoma
    B. Grave's disease
    C. Systemic lupus erythematosus
    D. Multiple sclerosis.

33. Which elevator muscle of the eyelid is involuntary?
    A. Levator palpebrae superioris
    B. Frontalis
    C. Muller's muscle
    D. Orbicularis oculi.

34. Fasanella Servat operation is indicated in:
    A. Congenital ptosis
    B. Traumatic ptosis
    C. Myasthenia gravis
    D. Horner's syndrome.

35. A patient with ptosis presents with retraction of the ptotic eyelid on chewing. This is called:
    A. Marcus Gunn jaw winking syndrome
    B. Third nerve misdirection syndrome
    C. Abducens palsy
    D. Oculomotor palsy.

36. Bilateral ptosis is not seen in:
    A. Marfan's syndrome
    B. Myasthenia gravis
    C. Myotonic dystrophy
    D. Kearns Sayre syndrome.

37. All of the following are potential side effects of edrophonium testing, except
    A. Tachycardia
    B. Respiratory arrest
    C. Syncope
    D. Vomitinh.

38. A patient diagnosed with myasthenia gravis (MG) requires:
    A. MRI scan of the brain
    B. B-scan ultrasonography of the eye and orbit
    C. CT scan of the chest
    D. Carotid Doppler ultrasonography.

39. Jaw winking is most commonly due to synkinesis of which two cranial nerves?
    A. Oculomotor and Facial
    B. Abducens and oculomotor
    C. Trigeminal and oculomotor
    D. Trochlear and abducens.

40. Eyelid synkinesis can occur in all of the following, except
    A. Congenital neurogenic blepharoptosis
    B. Ocular myasthenia gravis
    C. Aberrant nerve regeneration
    D. Duane retraction syndrome.

41. An early presentation of a 70 years old patient with involutional ptosis and good levator function is:
    A. Eyelid lag
    B. Supratarsal thickening
    C. Difficulty reading due to downgaze ptosis
    D. Unrelated to cataract surgery.

42. Chronic use of contact lenses results in ptosis due to:
    A. Involutional attenuation of the levator aponeurosis
    B. Repetitive eyelid traction
    C. Levator muscle dysgenesis
    D. Giant papillary conjunctivitis.

43. An infant presenting with a capillary hemangioma of the lid has which type of ptosis?
    A. Aponeurotic
    B. Mechanical
    C. Neurogenic
    D. Myogenic.

44. All of the following can be used in the treatment of the capillary hemangioma, except
    A. Dextromethorphan
    B. Propranolol
    C. Clobetasol propionate
    D. Interferon-α.

45. Before surgical repair, how long is it advised to observe traumatic ptosis in an adult?
    A. 4 weeks
    B. 2 months
    C. 6 months
    D. 12 months.

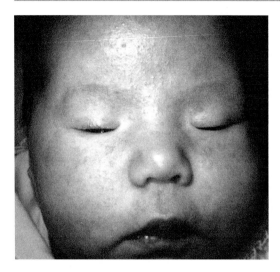

46. The systemic disorder most commonly associated with this disorder is:
    A. Diabetes mellitus
    B. Primary amenorrhea
    C. Hypospadias
    D. Coarctation of the aorta.

47. In patients with eyelid ptosis, which of the following is the most important measure in determining the type of surgery to perform?
    A. Margin reflex distance
    B. Levator function
    C. Response to phenylephrine testing
    D. Palpebral fissure width.

48. If one makes an incision 12 mm above the eyelid margin through the full thickness of the central upper eyelid, what is the correct order of the anatomic structures encountered?
    A. Skin, orbicularis oculi muscle, orbital septum, orbital fat, levator aponeurosis, Muller's muscle, conjunctiva
    B. Skin, orbital septum, orbicularis oculi muscle, orbital fat, levator aponeurosis, Muller's muscle, conjunctiva
    C. Skin, orbicularis oculi muscle, orbital septum, orbital fat, Muller's muscle, levator aponeurosis, conjunctiva
    D. Skin, orbicularis oculi muscle, orbital fat, orbital septum, levator aponeurosis, Muller's muscle, conjunctiva.

49. All of the following surgeries may be performed by making an incision at the lid crease except
    A. Blepharoplasty
    B. Fasanella Servat procedure
    C. Lateral orbitotomy
    D. Optic nerve sheath fenestration.

50. All of the following are true regarding the levator palpebrae superioris, except
    A. It runs from the posterior lacrimal crest medially to the lateral orbital tubercle laterally
    B. Its superficial portion inserts into the orbicularis muscle and subcutaneous tissues
    C. It originates in close proximity to the superior rectus origin, just above the annulus of Zinn.
    D. The muscular portion is shorter than the aponeurotic portion.

51. Components in the evaluation of corneal protective mechanisms prior to ptosis surgery include all of the following, except
    A. Examination for lagophthalmos
    B. Jones (primary dye) testing
    C. Assessment of Bell's phenomenon
    D. Evaluation of corneal sensation.

52. The primary abnormality seen in simple congenital ptosis is in the
    A. Levator muscle
    B. Levator aponeurosis
    C. Levator innervation
    D. Muller's muscle.

53. The primary abnormality seen in ptosis after cataract surgery is in the
    A. Levator muscle
    B. Levator aponeurosis
    C. Levator innervation
    D. Muller's muscle.

54. The procedure of choice in a patient with ptosis following cataract surgery would be
    A. Levator muscle resection
    B. Unilateral frontalis suspension

C. Muller's muscle resection
D. Reinsertion of levator aponeurosis.

55. Which is a clinical test specifically used in diagnosing myasthenia gravis (MG)?
   A. Exercise stress test
   B. Ice pack test
   C. Thyroid-stimulating hormone (TSH) receptor antibody test
   D. Three-step test.

56. In myogenic congenital ptosis, the levator complex (in the ptotic eye) is:
   A. Disinserted from the tarsus
   B. Histologically different from normal levator complex with decreased muscle fibers and fatty infiltrates
   C. Innervated by cranial nerve VII
   D. Absent below Whitnall ligament.

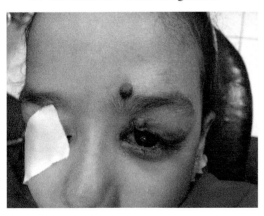

57. The above complication can occur with all materials used for frontalis suspension of *except*:
   A. Silicone
   B. Fascia lata
   C. Nylon (e.g., Supramid)
   D. Goretex.

58. Which of the following is not a component of Horner's syndrome?
   A. Miosis
   B. Anhidrosis
   C. Blepharoptosis
   D. Decreased stimulation of the levator muscle.

59. A 40-year-old patient is seen 2 months after blunt trauma to the right orbit. The examination is normal except for blepharoptosis on that side. Levator function is normal on both sides, and the patient states the eyelid positions were equal on both sides prior to the injury. There is no enophthalmos, and the patient does not complain of diplopia. What is the best next step in managing this patient?
   A. Surgical exploration and repair of the levator aponeurosis
   B. Close observation with no plan for surgical correction until 3–6 months after initial injury
   C. Computed tomography (CT) scan to rule out an orbital fracture
   D. A Tensilon test to rule out new-onset myasthenia gravis.

60. A patient with new onset ocular myasthenia gravis should have a chest CT scan done to look for what associated condition?
   A. Thymoma
   B. Sarcoid
   C. Apical lung tumor (Pancoast's tumor)
   D. Thyroid disease.

61. Which of the following is least useful in the evaluation of a patient with acquired ptosis?
   A. Interpalpebral fissures
   B. Frontalis muscle excursion
   C. Levator muscle function
   D. Margin-reflex distance.

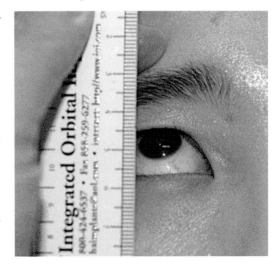

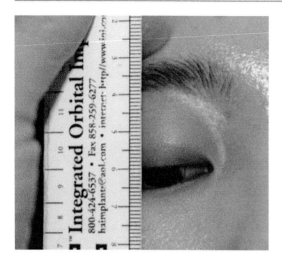

62. The patient is asked to look from extreme downgaze to extreme upgaze. What are you measuring?
    A. Levator muscle function
    B. Lid lag
    C. Lagophthalmos
    D. Muller's muscle function.

63. What is the most important measurement to use when deciding whether a frontalis sling is the preferred treatment for ptosis?
    A. Upper eyelid excursion
    B. Eyelid crease horizontal length
    C. Palpebral fissure
    D. Contralateral eyelid retraction.

64. A 75-year-old woman complains of restriction of her upper field of vision and difficulty reading when looking down. She denies any discomfort, epiphora, or diplopia. Her vision is J1+OU through her well-positioned bifocal segments. A basic tear secretion test is normal. Examination shows an eyelid malposition. What is the most likely diagnosis?
    A. Entropion
    B. Dermatochalasis
    C. Involutional ptosis
    D. Ectropion.

65. Recurrent unilateral, or bilateral, eyelid swelling in a younger patient is suggestive of which of the following diagnoses?
    A. Hemifacial spasm
    B. Gorlin's syndrome
    C. Dermatochalasis
    D. Blepharochalasis.

66. Which of the following is a contraindication to Muller's muscle conjunctival resection?
    A. Acquired aponeurogenic ptosis
    B. Post-cataract extraction ptosis
    C. No eyelid position change following instillation of topical phenylephrine
    D. Mild congenital ptosis.

67. Which of the following tests for myasthenia gravis can precipitate respiratory arrest?
    A. Tensilon test
    B. Acetylcholine receptor antibody titer
    C. Rest recovery
    D. Ice test.

68. A patient with congenital ptosis has bilateral measurements of margin reflex distance +1 mm, lid fissures of 5 mm, and lid excursions of 4 mm. What is the most appropriate surgical approach to treat the ptosis?
    A. Bilateral Mullerectomy
    B. Bilateral frontalis suspension
    C. Bilateral maximal external levator resection
    D. Bilateral Fasanella-Servat.

69. Which of the following signs is found in blepharochalasis syndrome?
    A. Cicatricial entropion
    B. Blepharoptosis
    C. Hypertrophy of orbital fat pads
    D. Thickened eyelid skin.

70. Regarding congenital myopathic ptosis, which is incorrect:
    A. Is less marked in downgaze
    B. Is associated with an indistinct or absent upper eyelid crease

C. Causes occlusive amblyopia in about 20% of patients

D. Is unilateral in about 70% of patients.

71. Regarding blepharophimosis syndrome, which is incorrect:
    A. Is always bilateral
    B. Also consists of telecanthus and epicanthus inversus
    C. Is commonly associated with mental retardation
    D. Is seen in 6% of children who have congenital ptosis.

72. Regarding Marcus Gunn jaw-winking, which is incorrect:
    A. Commonly involves the ipsilateral internal pterygoid muscle.
    B. Amplitude is greater in patients who have more severe ptosis.
    C. Often becomes less noticeable with increasing age.
    D. May require levator ablation as treatment.

73. Regarding dehiscence of the levator aponeurosis, which is incorrect:

    A. Is typically associated with poor levator function
    B. Is associated with an abnormally high or indistinct upper eyelid crease
    C. Occurs in 6% of patients after cataract surgery
    D. May be caused by contact lens wear.

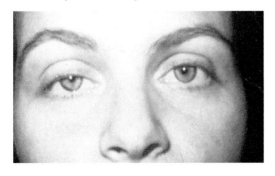

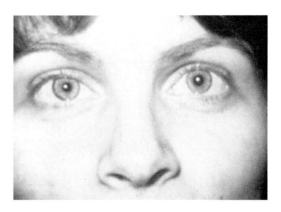

74. The above 42 years old myopic patient has been using contact lenses for 15 years. The most probable surgical procedure used to correct her ptosis was:
    A. Bilateral levator muscle resection
    B. Bilateral levator aponeurosis reinsertion
    C. Bilateral Muller muscle resection
    D. Bilateral frontalis sling.

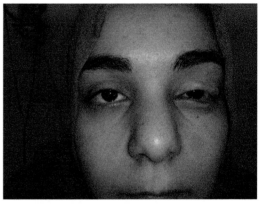

75. Causes of this complication following ptosis surgery include all except:
    A. Extensive use of diathermy
    B. Extensive dissection around the root of the lashes
    C. Extensive dissection on the posterior surface of the levator
    D. Extensive dissection on the anterior surface of the levator.

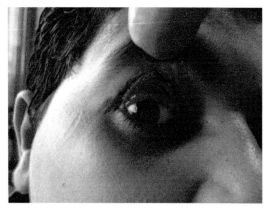

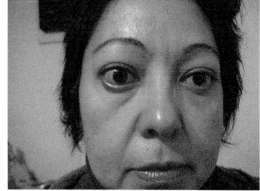

76. This complication following ptosis surgery occurs due to:
    A. Extensive use of diathermy
    B. Extensive dissection around the root of the lashes
    C. Extensive dissection on the posterior surface of the levator
    D. Extensive dissection on the anterior surface of the levator.

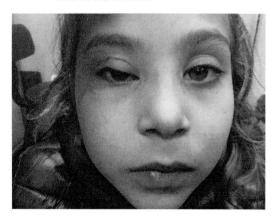

77. This complication of ptosis surgery can be prevented by:
    A. Use of local anesthesia with intraoperative adjustment
    B. Use of 3 sutures for muscle fixation
    C. Proper dissection of both muscle horns
    D. Complete opening of the orbital septum.

78. This complication of ptosis surgery can be prevented by:
    A. Use of local anesthesia with intraoperative adjustment
    B. Use of 3 sutures for muscle fixation
    C. Proper dissection of both muscle horns
    D. Complete opening of the orbital septum.

79. Advantages of frontalis flap procedure includes all except:
    A. No risk of rejection or severe body reaction
    B. The flap grows with the child
    C. The flap develops before fascia lata
    D. Presence of a remote but acceptable scar.

80. Frontalis flap procedure results in all except:
    A. Less lid lag on downgaze
    B. Less ptosis on upgaze
    C. Preservation of lid contour
    D. Progressive cheese-wiring effect.

81. Indications of frontalis flap include all except:
    A. Acquired ptosis with poor levator function
    B. Congenital ptosis with poor levator function
    C. Recurrent cases after levator surgery
    D. Traumatic ptosis with forehead scars.

82. Regarding the surgical technique for frontalis flap procedure, which is false:
    A. Requires a long learning curve
    B. Is adjustable
    C. Can be done through a single incision
    D. Is essentially a rotational flap.

83. The following drops can improve the ptosis temporarily except:
    A. Apraclonidine
    B. Oxymetazoline
    C. Naphazoline
    D. Phenyepherine.

84. Which of the following is associated with type 2 blepharophimosis syndrome?
    A. Epicanthus tarsalis
    B. Gene mutation in *FOXL2*
    C. Primary ovarian failure
    D. Increased interpupillary distance.

Answers for this chapter ptosis

1	B	21	D	41	C	61	A	81	D
2	C	22	C	42	B	62	A	82	A
3	A	23	A	43	B	63	A	83	C
4	C	24	B	44	A	64	C	84	B
5	B	25	A	45	C	65	D		
6	B	26	D	46	B	66	C		
7	B	27	B	47	B	67	A		
8	C	28	C	48	A	68	B		
9	B	29	D	49	B	69	B		
10	D	30	D	50	D	70	C		
11	B	31	A	51	B	71	C		
12	C	32	D	52	A	72	A		
13	C	33	C	53	B	73	A		
14	B	34	D	54	D	74	C		
15	A	35	A	55	B	75	C		
16	B	36	A	56	B	76	C		
17	B	37	A	57	B	77	B		
18	A	38	C	58	D	78	A		
19	B	39	C	59	B	79	D		
20	B	40	B	60	A	80	D		

Lid Reconstruction

4

Essam A. El Toukhy

Traumatic and post-surgical eyelid defects vary in size, complexity, and amount of tissue loss. An extensive knowledge of the anatomy of the ocular adnexa and potential options for repair allows the surgeon to individually tailor the reconstruction to best suit the patients' needs. This chapter provides a highlight of multiple useful approaches for varying degrees of eyelid reconstruction.

The pre-operative consultation for eyelid reconstruction is central to surgical success and centers around managing patient expectations. It should address potential functional and cosmetic outcomes as well as potential for additional surgical interventions. Small lesions can end up with unexpectedly large defects being 'tip of the iceberg' phenomenon. With proper reconstruction, lid tissues will usually reach excellent healing over 6–12 months in the vast majority of cases. Procedures of the nasolacrimal system must be addressed including silicone intubation or the possibility of future conjunctivo-dacryocystorhinostomy if sacrifice of the canaliculi is required. Similarly, globe prominence, hypoplasticity of the inferior orbital rim, eyelid laxity, and actinic damage should all be addressed.

Assessment of patient comorbidities, medications and allergies is an important portion of the preoperative evaluation. Anticoagulation should be stopped in the perioperative period whenever reasonable with respect to the patients' systemic risks and with the permission of the prescribing physician.

The goals of tumor excision and reconstruction should be outlined in order of importance: Removal of the malignancy; restoration of function; cosmesis.

Defects of the anterior lamella of the eyelid can be repaired by direct closure, rotational flaps, grafts, or a combination of these methods. The targeted repair of the posterior and anterior lamellae with careful attention on the amount of tension results in improved post-operative function and cosmesis. This reconstruction serves as the backbone for many of the repairs

- Reconstruction of both the anterior and posterior lamellae are required
- Either the anterior or posterior lamella must have a blood supply
- A graft on top of a graft will result in failure of both grafts
- A pedicle flap is required for one of the lamellae
- Minimize vertical tension on the eyelid during closure
- Horizontal tension will typically improve with healing
- Vertical tension will not and will cause eyelid malposition

E. A. El Toukhy (✉)
Oculoplasty Service, Cairo University, Cairo, Egypt
e-mail: eeltoukhy@yahoo.com

E. A. El Toukhy (ed.), *Oculoplasty for Ophthalmologists*, https://doi.org/10.1007/978-3-030-68469-3_4

- Match tissue color, texture, and quality as best possible
- Limit cautery to the minimal required amount
- Anatomic re-creation of the canthi is paramount to achieve a stable lid
- Use of a frost suture to prevent early postoperative retraction and to protect the globe during healing.

A detailed description of the use and steps of lid reconstruction techniques are covered in this chapter.

Lid Reconstruction:

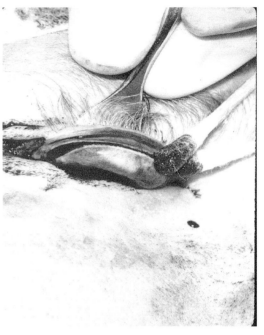

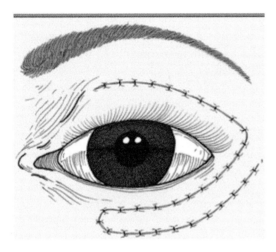

1. The above technique is ideal in:
   A. Lower Lid coloboma
   B. Lower lid retaction
   C. Lower lid benign lesions
   D. Lower lid malignant lesions.

2. The above technique is ideal in:
   A. Lower Lid coloboma
   B. Lower lid retaction
   C. Lower lid benign lesions
   D. Lower lid malignant lesions.

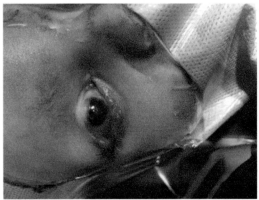

3. This lesion is:
   A. Traumatic
   B. Congenital
   C. Inflammatory
   D. Neoplastic.

4. When planning reconstruction of an eyelid defect the surgeon should:
   A. Replace both anterior and posterior lamella with grafts
   B. Avoid undermining adjacent tissue
   C. Minimize vertical tension
   D. Allow wound to granulate prior to reconstruction.

5. Regarding congenital coloboma the most appropriate statement is:
   A. An isolated anomaly if present in the upper medial eyelid
   B. Eyelid margin is not involved
   C. Distichiasis is not a feature of this disease
   D. Eyelid sharing procedures are recommended for children.

6. After surgical excision of a lower lid tumor, the most appropriate procedure for moderate defect (<50%) is:
   A. Semicircular advancement or rotation flaps
   B. Advancement of a transconjunctival flap from the upper eyelid into the posterior lamellar defect
   C. Mustarde procedure
   D. Free transconjunctival autografts from the upper eyelid.

7. Congenital colobomas of the eyelids are associated with which systemic syndrome?
   A. Goldenhar's syndrome
   B. Pierre Robin's syndrome
   C. Hallermann-Streiff syndrome
   D. Stickler's syndrome.

8. A 60-year-old patient underwent full thickness surgical excision of a squamous cell carcinoma that occupied half of the upper eyelid. Which of the following procedures is best suited for her eyelid reconstruction?
   A. Direct closure with lateral canthotomy
   B. Tenzel semicircular flap
   C. Cutler-Beard procedure
   D. Hughes procedure.

9. Which of the following is not a good option for full thickness skin grafting:
   A. Upper eyelid skin
   B. Retroauricular
   C. Preauricular
   D. Hard palate.

10. In lid reconstruction; one can use all except:
    A. A flap for the anterior lamella and a flap for the posterior lamella
    B. A flap for the anterior lamella and a graft for the posterior lamella
    C. A graft for the anterior lamella and a flap for the posterior lamella
    D. A graft for the anterior lamella and a graft for the posterior lamella.

11. A young male with a history of eyelid trauma was seeking lid reconstruction after primary repair, during surgery we should avoid all except;
    A. Replacing both anterior and posterior lamellae with grafts
    B. Excising adjacent tissue
    C. Vertical tension
    D. Horizontal tension.
    This 60% defect resulted after a Mohs surgical procedure

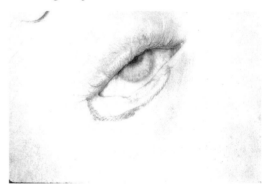

12. What surgical method would be the most appropriate for reconstruction of the posterior lamella?
    A. Cutler-Beard flap
    B. Bipedicle myocutaneous flap
    C. Full-thickness skin graft
    D. Hughes tarsoconjunctival flap.

13. What is the *least* likely cause that led to the eyelid defect?
    A. Basal cell carcinoma
    B. Metastatic cancer
    C. Sebaceous cell carcinoma
    D. Squamous cell carcinoma.

14. A recurrent squamous cell carcinoma is excised from the medial canthus. Which of the following reconstructive techniques should be avoided to prevent detection of a deep delayed recurrence?
    A. Midforehead rotational flap
    B. Full thickness skin graft from the retro-auricular area
    C. Full thickness skin graft from the upper eyelid
    D. Undermining with direct closure.

15. Excisional biopsy is a useful treatment modality in which of the following?
    A. Lattice corneal dystrophy
    B. Ocular cicatricial pemphigoid
    C. Nodular scleritis
    D. Conjunctival intraepithelial neoplasia.

16. What is the most common complication following repair of total eyelid defects (upper and lower)?
    A. Need for dacryocystorhinostomy
    B. Eyelid rigidity manifested by ptosis and lagophthalmos
    C. Proptosis
    D. Corneal ulceration.

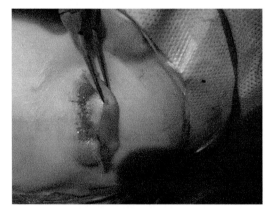

17. This technique is:
    A. Hughes flap
    B. Semicircular flap
    C. Cutler Beard flap
    D. Mustarde flap.

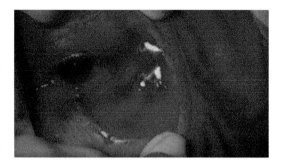

18. This lid defect requires:
    A. Hughes flap and a skin graft
    B. Semicircular flap and a skin graft
    C. Cutler Beard flap and a skin graft
    D. Mustarde flap and a skin graft.

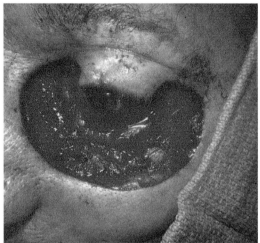

19. This defect requires:
    A. Hughes flap and a skin graft
    B. Semicircular flap and a skin graft
    C. Cutler Beard flap and a skin graft
    D. Mustarde flap and a skin graft.

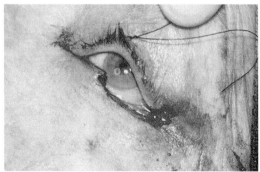

20. The best choice for this defect is:
    A. Hughes flap with two stage reconstruction
    B. A tarso conjunctival transposition flap
    C. A hard palate graft
    D. A Mustarde flap and a skin graft.

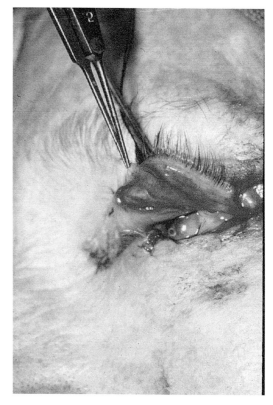

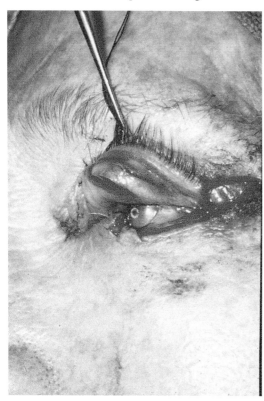

21. The advantages of this technique include all except:
    A. Maintaining two point fixation
    B. Single stage procedure
    C. Does not require a skin graft
    D. Lined by mucous membrane.

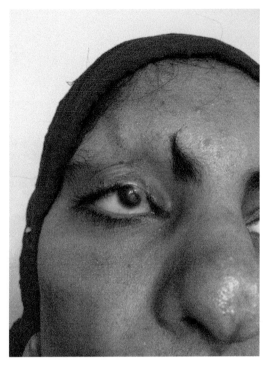

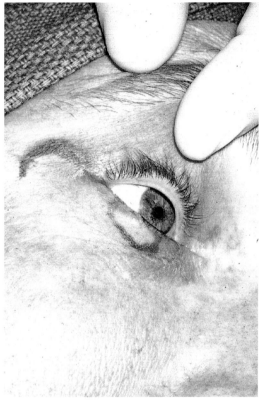

22. All are true regarding the above lesion except:
    A. Requires staged reconstruction
    B. Requires mucous membrane graft from the lip or palate
    C. No need for lid sharing
    D. The brow defect can be repaired simultaneously.

23. The height of the semicircular defect equals:
    A. Up 33% of the lid margin
    B. Up to 50% of the lid margin
    C. The width of the defect
    D. The length of the defect.

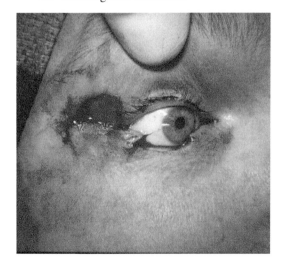

24. The next step in the surgical technique is:
    A. Cutting the capsulopalpebral fascia
    B. Release of the orbital septum
    C. Cutting the lateral palpebral ligament
    D. Creating a periosteal flap.

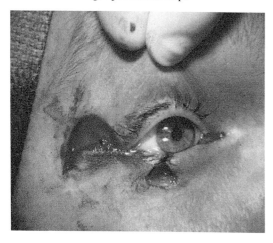

25. The next step in the surgical technique is:
    A. Lid margin repair
    B. Creating two point fixation
    C. Closure of deep tissues
    D. Reforming the lateral canthus.

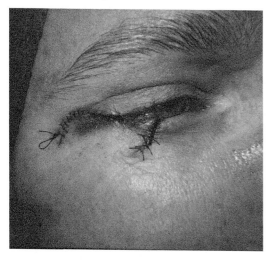

26. The advantages of this technique include all except:
    A. Maintaining two point fixation
    B. Single stage procedure
    C. Leaving a noticeable scar
    D. Lined by mucous membrane.

27. In the repair of a total eyelid defect from trauma, what is the preferred use of the avulsed tissue?
    A. Reimplantation even if the tissue has been ischemic for several hours
    B. Avoidance of reimplantation because of infection potential
    C. Avoidance of reimplantation because of graft-versus-host disease
    D. Reimplantation with chemotherapy.
28. The below technique is used for:
    A. Lower lid Entropion
    B. Lower lid Ectropion
    C. Lower lid retraction
    D. Lower lid Laxity.

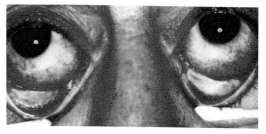

29. In lid reconstruction; "Two Point Fixation" means:
    A. Suturing both the orbicularis muscle and levator muscle
    B. Recreation of the medial and lateral canthal tendons
    C. Suturing both lids together and creating a temporary tarsorraphy at the end of the procedure
    D. Adjusting the eyelid contour medially and laterally.

Answers of Lid Reconstruction

1	B	11	D	21	C
2	D	12	D	22	B
3	B	13	B	23	C
4	C	14	A	24	C
5	A	15	D	25	B
6	A	16	B	26	C
7	A	17	C	27	A
8	C	18	A	28	C
9	D	19	A	29	B
10	D	20	B		

Cosmetics and Injectables

Noha El Toukhy

Facial rejuvenation encompasses correction of facial rhytides and volume attrition by cosmetic surgical or non-surgical procedures. Facial ageing is an ongoing natural process which is influenced by intrinsic and extrinsic factors. The synergistic effects of reduction of tissue elasticity, collagen loss, soft tissue atrophy, persistent use of facial muscles and the effects of gravity are the main factors for the intrinsic tissue changes. Photo degradation of tissues, smoking, lifestyle habits are some of the extrinsic contributors. The fundamental principle of facial rejuvenation is to reverse or hault these changes with surgical or non surgical methods to improve the tissue descent, restore the lost volume, and improve the quality of the skin.

Cosmetic rejuvenation of the periocular area can include incisional and non-incisional procedures. Although the use of non-incisional procedures, including botulinum toxin, dermal fillers, and skin resurfacing, has gained in popularity, the oculoplastic surgeon should continue to be proficient in incisional procedures. The most common periocular incisional procedures include upper blepharoplasty, lower blepharoplasty, mid-face lift and browplasty. Careful preoperative evaluation is critical, and the choice of the appropriate surgery is paramount.

Cosmetic upper blepharoplasty involves the removal or skin, orbicularis muscle, and/or fat of the upper lid. Patients' complaints usually involve an extra fold of skin or puffiness of the upper eyelid. Lateral lacrimal gland prolapse should be noted, and if present, should be addressed during the surgery with repositioning of the gland. The brow and upper lid constitute a continuum which must be evaluated in any patient undergoing an upper lid blepharoplasty.

As in the upper eyelid, the skin of the lower eyelid is the thinnest in the body and is devoid of subcutaneous fat. Aging changes in the lower eyelid occur variably in each patient: tear trough deformity, orbital fat prolapse, loss of skin elasticity, or orbicularis prominence. A customized approach considering each patient's lower eyelid configuration is important. Surgical procedures for lower blepharoplasty include the transcutaneous approach and the transconjunctival approach. Fat can be removed or repositioned into depressed region. The lower eyelids have several particularly subtle anatomical and functional considerations that the careful surgeon must consider to select the appropriate approach. Overlooking small variations in anatomy and function can lead to suboptimal outcomes or complications in lower eyelid surgery. Proper planning and exact execution are essential to have a good surgical outcome in performing lower blepharoplasty.

N. El Toukhy (✉)
Haverford College, Haverford, PA, USA
e-mail: nohaelt@yahoo.com

© The Author(s), under exclusive license to Springer Nature Switzerland AG 2021
E. A. El Toukhy (ed.), *Oculoplasty for Ophthalmologists*, https://doi.org/10.1007/978-3-030-68469-3_5

As the lower eyelid transitions to the cheek inferiorly, the suborbicularis oculi fat pad (SOOF) is deep to the orbital orbicularis oculi over the inferior orbital rim. Inferior to the rim, the superficial musculoaponeurotic system (SMAS) overlies the SOOF. Superficial to the SMAS lies an additional malar fat pad. The correct position of both the SOOF and the malar fat pad lead to a high, smooth cheek characteristic of the youthful midface.

For the lower lids; Preoperative clinical evaluations must address all of the following: Skin laxity and wrinkles, Fat prolapse, Tear trough deformity, Eyelid position, Eyelid laxity. Techniques include: Transcutaneous lower blepharoplasty, Lateral tarsal strip, lateral SMAS lifting, Transconjunctival lower blepharoplasty, Subtractive blepharoplasty, tissue redraping (fat repositioning) blepharoplasty and Pinch technique skin excision.

Injectables offer an excellent non-surgical method of facial rejuvenation. Among which, botulinum toxin (BTX) and soft tissue fillers are one of the most common and favorite tools for non-surgical rejuvenation.

BTX injections, frequently applied in treating spastic facial dystonias have been used for decades and are still the most preferable treatment methods today due to undesired effects of alternative treatment methods.

In addition to being used to reduce wrinkles, BTX is successfully used in the temporary treatment of idiopathic and thyroid dysfunction induced upper eyelid retraction, inoperable lacrimal duct blockage and temporary induction of ptosis in facial paralysis, as well as in other areas including extremity hyperhidrosis, bruxism, migraine, tension-type headaches, and paralytic spasticity. BTX injections to minimize scar formation have also been reported.

Its effect on wrinkles has an early temporary reversible phase with relaxation of the muscle tone and decreased force of contraction giving a better appearance during animation. With repeated injections, the late permanent stable phase results in remodeling of the dermis and skin to achieve a lasting improvement. So, in addition to decreasing wrinkles that are present, ultimately, prolonged use of BTX prevents further deepening of the crease and truly prevents signs of aging. Best response is seen in ages between 30–50 years. The effects of Botox are cumulative, and results improve on repeated treatment.

As a cosmetic agent, Botulinum toxin has been used in the management of: forehead wrinkles, glabellar folds (frown lines), lower lid wrinkles, crow's feet, orbicularis hypertrophy (sausage roll orbicularis), brow lift and repositioning, upper gum show (gummy smile), vertical lip lines (smoking lines), mental crease and notch, masseter injection (Texas jaw line), vertical platysmal bands. And recently, the introduction of the mesobotox technique and the Baby Botox technique.

Fillers are substances used for augmentation of soft tissues or fill up the volume attrition due to subcutaneous fat loss associated with aging. With increasing age, the body's natural potential to produce hyaluronic acid as well as its inherent hygroscopy decreases thereby playing an important role in facial soft tissue atrophy. Fillers are primarily indicated for volume augmentation and correction of static rhytides. They restore symmetry and the volume loss on the face. Soft tissue fillers help in re-augmentation of the depleting collagen, and support and lift the fat pads and ligaments. The role of dermal fillers for facial aesthetics has been revolutionised with the introduction of Hyaluronic acid (HA) fillers. The newer Hyaluronic Acid (HA) based agents have restored the interest in dermal fillers as they promise better outcomes with a lesser side effect.

Fillers are an excellent adjunct to botulinum toxin and in many cases, the combination is superior to surgery. An ideal combination is the administration of the neurotoxin to relax the muscles of facial expression and maximally reduce the dynamic lines, and subsequently, a filler is injected to further reduce any remaining static lines.

Some of the common indications for its use are:

1. Upper face: correction of glabellar lines, superior sulcus deformity, temporal fossa hollowing and forehead contouring
2. Mid- face: midface lift, correction of tear trough deformity, cheek augmentation, nose augmentation and contouring
3. Lower face: lip augmentation, marionette lines, perioral rhytides, downturned oral commissures, and irregular chin lines, pre-jowl sulcus, redefining of jaw line and chin augmentation.

The number of patients with body dysmorphic disorder, a mental disorder where patients spend the majority of their time worrying about slight or un-noticeable flaws in their appearances, has greatly increased over the past decades. It is important to understand that patients struggling with BDD are in need of psychological assistance, not surgical help. These patients do not need surgeries, but instead, should be referred to psychologists, who would work on the patients' sense of self perception and self-esteem.

Cosmetics & injectables

1. Botulinum toxin is indicated in all the following except:
   A. Lid retraction
   B. Entropion
   C. Ectropion
   D. Aberrant regeneration of cranial nerves.
2. Botulinum toxin is indicated in all the following except:
   A. Irreparable lacrimal obstruction
   B. Crocodile tears syndroms
   C. Tension headache
   D. Migraine headache.
3. Botulinum toxin is indicated in all the following except:
   A. Healing of facial wounds
   B. Lagophthalmos due to facial palsy
   C. Ptosis
   D. Wrinkle improvement.

4. Complications of Botulinum toxin injections include all except:
   A. Ectropion
   B. Ptosis
   C. Epiphora
   D. Lid lag.
5. Complications of Botulinum toxin injections include all except:
   A. Diplopia
   B. Dermatochalasis
   C. Lagophthalmos
   D. Gum show.
6. Ptosis caused by Botulinum injection can be partly reversed by
   A. Carbonic anhydrase inhibitors
   B. Prostaglandin analogues
   C. B- blockers
   D. Alpha-agonists.
7. Brow Ptosis can be treated by all except :
   A. Surgery
   B. Endoscopy
   C. Injections
   D. Laser.
8. The upper lid has how many pre-aponeurotic fat pads?:
   A. One
   B. Two
   C. Three
   D. Four.
9. The lower lid has how many pre-aponeurotic fat pads?:
   A. One
   B. Two
   C. Three
   D. Four.
10. All the following drugs should be stopped before blepharoplasty except:
    A. Herbal supplements
    B. Aspirin
    C. Antihypertensives
    D. Steroids.

11. Regarding periocular Botulinum toxin injections , one is false:
    A. Onabotulinum toxin A was the first toxin available for aesthetic indications
    B. Is the treatment of choice for benign essential blepharospasm
    C. Duration of effect is typically 12 months
    D. Complications includes ptosis and corneal exposures.

12 Soft tissue dermal fillers , one is false:
    A. Bovine collagen filler was the first filler
    B. The hyaluronic acid fillers were derived from bacteria
    C. The hyaluronic acid fillers requires skin testing for allergic reaction before use
    D. Complication of periocular fillers injection includes central retinal artery occlusion.

13. True statement regarding benign essential blepharospasm:
    A. Unilateral focal dystonia
    B. More common in males
    C. Muscles of the face are also involved
    D. Caused by vascular compression of the facial nerve.

14. Regarding laser lid skin resurfacing, one is false
    A. Ultrapulsed CO_2 and Erbium YAG laser are the most widely used
    B. Ultrapulsed CO_2 laser has a small thermal injury into the tissue than Erbium YAG laser
    C. The darker the skin pigmentation , the greater the risk of postoperative inflammation
    D. Herpes simplex virus infection after laser resurfacing is associated with scaring.

15. Few hours following blepharoplasty, the patient complains of pain and reduced vision noticed to have proptosis and abnormal pupillary reaction, the most appropriate step is:
    A. CT scan.
    B. Canthotomy and cantholysis to release retro orbital hemorrhage.

C. IV steroids for compressive optic neuropathy.
D. Observation and pain management.

16. Regarding botulinum toxin, one of the following statement is true:
    A. Used in blepharospasm.
    B. Must be avoided in patient with hemifacial spam due to risk of brain aneurysm.
    C. Lid retraction is a known side effect.
    D. Botulinum toxin B used in cosmetic wrinkle reduction.

17. Hemifacial spasm is usually associated with all of the following except:
    A. Bilaterality
    B. Age of onset over 50 years
    C. Vascular etiology
    D. Involuntary spasm of the orbicularis muscle.

18. Few hours following bilateral blepharoplasty a patient complain of sudden pain near the left eye. Removal of the dressing and local examination reveals tense and ecchymotic left eyelids. The first step would be in the management of this case:
    A. Treatment with ice packs
    B. Visual acuity measurement and check pupillary responses
    C. Check corneal sensation for a possibility of a cavernous sinus thrombosis
    D. Open the wound to release a possible retrobulbar hemorrhage.

19. When performing mid-face rejuvenation which structure is elevated to its previous anatomic position?
    A. Preseptal orbicularis
    B. Retro-orbicularis oculi fat
    C. Lateral canthal tendon
    D. Suborbicularis oculi fat (SOOF).

20. Botulinum toxin is indicated in all the following except:
    A. Essential blepharospasm
    B. Postoperative residual squint

C. A-pattern exotropia
D. Hemifacial spasm.

21. Complications of Upper blepharoplasty include all except:
   A. Ptosis
   B. Lid retraction
   C. Lagophthalmos
   D. Ectropion.

22. Complications of Upper blepharoplasty include all except:
   A. Orbital hemorrhage
   B. Asymmetry
   C. Brow ptosis
   D. Lid gangrene.

23. Complications of Upper blepharoplasty include all except:
   A. Dry eyes
   B. Scar formation
   C. Infection
   D. Entropion.

24. Regarding lacrimal gland prolapse:
   A. Is a frequent finding in dermatochalasis
   B. Will disappear after upper blepharoplasty
   C. Requires excision
   D. Requires a separate procedure later.

25. Regarding tear trough deformity, all are true except:
   A. Is due to descent of the SOOF and malar fat pads
   B. Requires volume addition
   C. Results in a double convexity appearance
   D. Can only be corrected surgically.

26. Preoperative evaluation of the lower lids before blepharoplasty should include all except:
   A. SOOF position
   B. SMAS position
   C. Puntal position
   D. Lacrimal gland position.

27. Preoperative evaluation of the lower lids before blepharoplasty should include all except:
   A. Skin laxity
   B. Tear trough
   C. Eyelid laxity
   D. Eyelid excursion.

28. Preoperative evaluation of the lower lids before blepharoplasty should include all except:
   A. Snap back test
   B. Distraction test
   C. Jones test
   D. Fat distribution.

29. The pinch technique is used to determine:
   A. Site of incision
   B. Amount of skin resected
   C. Amount of orbicularis resected
   D. Amount of fat resected.

30. Regarding persistant conjunctival chemosis following blepharoplasty, all are true except:
   A. Requires pressure bandage
   B. Is caused mainly by lymphatic obstruction
   C. May need surgical excision
   D. Occurs more in diabetics.

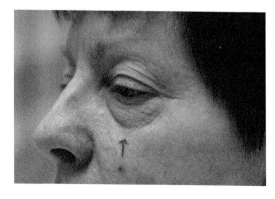

31. Cosmetic correction of the above lid can be done by all except:
   A. Botox injections
   B. Transcutaneous blepharoplasty
   C. Fat repositioning
   D. Lower lid tightening procedure.

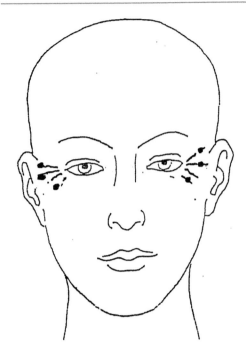

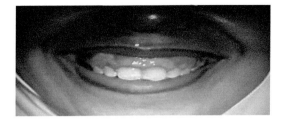

34. Treatment of this cosmetic complaint requires Botox injection in which muscle:
    A. Orbicularis Oris
    B. Buccinator
    C. Levator labii superioris
    D. Levator anguli oris.

32. Botox injection in this area can result in all except:
    A. Ptosis
    B. Diplopia
    C. Brow elevation
    D. Epiphora.

35. In the midface, botox has all the following effects except:
    A. Eliminate gummy smile
    B. Eliminate smoking lines
    C. Induce Texas jaw line
    D. Induce mental crease.

36. The " baby Botox " technique entails all except:
    A. Injection in younger patients
    B. Injection of smaller doses
    C. Injection more frequently
    D. Less stability of results.

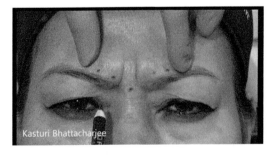

37. Fillers are used in the cosmetic correction of all except:
    A. Superior sulcus deformity
    B. Tear trough deformity
    C. Depressed scars
    D. Sausage shaped orbicularis.

33. Botox injection in this area can result in all except:
    A. Ptosis
    B. Central retinal artery occlusion
    C. Brow elevation
    D. Diplopia.

38. Fillers are used in the cosmetic correction of all except:
    A. Lower lid wrinkles
    B. Upper lid wrinkles
    C. Cheek augmentation
    D. Periorbital hyperpigmentation.

39. Patients with body dysmorphic disorder (BDD) have:
    a. Type A personality
    b. Obvious cosmetic body defect
    c. History of multiple surgeries
    d. Unrealistic expectations.

40. Management of body dysmorphic disordere requires:
    A. Proper preoperative identification
    B. Use of special assessment tools and questionnaires
    C. Referal to psychologists
    D. A clear plan for surgery.

41. Regarding blepharoplasty , one is false:
    A. Lower lid blepharoplasty is most commonly performed for cosmetic indications
    B. Upper lid blepharoplasty is most commonly performed for functional reasons
    C. Difficulty in reading is an indication for functional lower lid blepharoplasty
    D. Cosmetic upper lid blepharoplasty often requires skin rejuvenation and chemical peals.

42. Regarding blepharoplasty techniques , one is false:
    A. Transconjunctival incision is preferred more than subciliary incision in lower lid blepharoplasty
    B. At least 20 mm of skin should remain between the inferior border of the eye brow and the lower eye lid margin in upper lid blepharoplasty
    C. During blepharoplasty surgery in a patient with dry eye syndrome ,the surgeon should preserve orbicularis oculi muscle
    D. The amount of excess skin to be excised is determined by pinch technique.

43. Complication of blepharoplasty surgery , one is false:
    A. Loss of vision usually associated with lower lid blepharoplasty more than upper lid

    B. TED is regarded as a risk factor for post blepharoplasty surgery orbital hemorrhage
    C. Pressure dressing should be conducted directly after surgery
    D. Urgent orbital decompression then high dose of IV steroid is the management of choice for postoperative orbital hemorrhage.

44. Essential blepharospasm is usually characterized by all of the following except:
    A. Unilaterality.
    B. Age of onset usually over 50 years.
    C. Obscure etiology
    D. Involuntary spasm of the orbicularis muscle.

45. Rhytidectomy refers to:
    A. Face lift
    B. Brow lift
    C. Laser skin resurfacing
    D. Injection of botox.

46. A patient calls to report pain, sudden swelling, and decreased vision the night after a blepharoplasty procedure. What should be done?
    A. Advise the patient to use ice packs to decrease the swelling.
    B. Set up an appointment for the patient to see you the next day.
    C. Make arrangements to see the patient as soon as possible.
    D. Reassure the patient that discomfort, swelling, and blurry vision are normal postoperative findings.

47. Which one of the following statements regarding blepharoplasty is FALSE?
    A. Repair of lower eyelid dermatochalasis and / or steatoblepharon may be followed by lower eyelid retraction.
    B. A transconjunctival blepharoparoplasty is a procedure primarily used to perform upper eyelid surgery when trying to avoid an anterior incision.

C. The advantage of eyelid crease fixation in conjunction with blepharoplasty is that it aligns the eyelid crease and the postoperative scar.

D. Damage to the inferior oblique muscle is a potential complication of both anterior and posterior approaches to lower eyelid blepharoplasty.

48. The following are true about the preaponeurotic fat EXCEPT:
    A. It is situated between the orbital septum and the levator
    B. The trochlea divides the fat into a medial and a lateral pad
    C. The medial pad has more fibrous tissue than the lateral pad
    D. The medial pad has a yellowish appearance whereas the lateral pad is white.

49. The following are true about the orbital septum EXCEPT:
    A. Is attached to the arcus marginalis of the orbital rim
    B. Is inserted on the levator at point where the levator muscle becomes aponeurosis
    C. Is attached to the retractors 4mm below the inferior tarsal border
    D. Limits the spread of cellulitis into the orbit.

50. All of the following favor the diagnosis of benign essential blepharospasm over hemifacial spasm, except
    A. Absence of abnormal movements during sleep.
    B. No involvement of lower facial muscles.
    C. Synchronous contractures of involved muscles.
    D. Lack of response to neurosurgical decompression of the facial nerve.

51. What preoperative medication is most appropriate for reducing the chance of irreversible scarring in patients prior to undergoing laser skin resurfacing?
    A. Valacyclovir.
    B. Prednisone.
    C. Diphenhydramine.
    D. Mitomycin-C.

52. Laser skin resurfacing is contraindicated in patients taking which one of the following medications?
    A. Isotretinoin.
    B. Hydrochlorothiazide.
    C. Docetaxel.
    D. Sildenafil citrate.

53. The most likely outcome following inadvertent suturing of the orbital septum into subcutaneous tissues while performing blepharoplasty is
    A. Ectropion.
    B. Lid retraction in downgaze.
    C. Entropion.
    D. Blepharoptosis.

54. All of the following are characteristic of features of blepharochalasis, except
    A. Lacrimal gland atrophy.
    B. Excess eyelid skin.
    C. Blepharoptosis.
    D. Blepharophimosis.

55. Which of the following extraocular muscles is least likely to be injured during upper or lower blepharoplasty?
    A. Inferior oblique.
    B. Inferior rectus.
    C. Superior oblique.
    D. Superior rectus.

56. The most significant complication of blepharoplasty is
    A. Orbital hemorrhage.
    B. Diplopia.
    C. Overcorrection.
    D. Cellulitis.

57. The carbon dioxide laser has all of the following characteristics *except:*
    A. Wavelength in the infrared spectrum
    B. Able to be seen by the human eye
    C. Utilized for orbital tumor excision
    D. Operates at 10.6 μm

58. The site of action of botulinum toxin type A (Botox), when used to treat facial movement disorders, is the:
    A. Motor nerve terminal, inhibiting acetylcholine release
    B. Motor nerve terminal, promoting cholinesterase release
    C. Plasma membrane (sarcolemma) of the striated muscle, inhibiting acetylcholine release
    D. Plasma membrane (sarcolemma) of the striated muscle, promoting cholinesterase release

59. What is the most common complication of external lower eyelid blepharoplasty?
    A. Lower eyelid retraction
    B. Pyogenic granuloma at the incision site
    C. Lash loss
    D. Bacterial infection at the incision site

60. A patient is evaluated preoperatively for blepharoplasty surgery. Which of the following is not a relative contraindication to surgery?
    A. Poorly controlled hypertension
    B. Severe keratoconjunctivitis sicca
    C. Insulin-dependent diabetes
    D. Atrial fibrillation with anticoagulation.

61. A young girl has had transitory bilateral, painless eyelid edema which lasts over years. There is no history of erythema, pruritus, or atopy. Examination shows baggy upper eyelid skin with a crepe paper-like appearance. For this patient, what is the most likely diagnosis?
    A. Contact dermatitis
    B. Thyroid eye disease
    C. Dermatochalasis
    D. Blepharochalasis.

62. A young patient presents with a high forehead and brow ptosis. Which of the following is the best surgical approach to treat the brow ptosis?
    A. Pretrichial endoscopic forehead lift
    B. Coronal forehead lift

C. Direct eyebrow elevation
D. Midforehead lift.

63. For what type of facial spasm is magnetic resonance imaging useful?
    A. Hemifacial spasm
    B. Benign essential blepharospasm
    C. Acute facial nerve palsy followed by aberrant regeneration
    D. Blepharospasm associated with dry eyes.

64. Complications of blepharoplasty include all except:
    A. Superior rectus muscle weakness.
    B. Epiphora.
    C. Lower lid retraction.
    D. Ptosis.

65. Regarding laser skin resurfacing, which is incorrect:
    A. Should be avoided in keloid-forming patients.
    B. Can eliminate wrinkles and skin imperfections.
    C. Gives best results in patients who have fair complexions.
    D. May cause reactivation of herpes simplex.

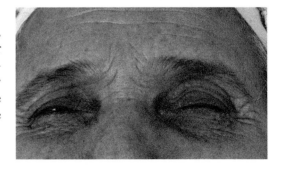

66. Regarding the above disorder, which is incorrect:
    A. Usually occurs in patients older than 50 years.
    B. May be associated with phenothiazine use.
    C. Is not associated with familial dystonia.
    D. Is usually bilateral.

67. In severe cases of essential blepharospasm, one may see all except:
    A. Decreased tear production.
    B. Brow ptosis.
    C. Ectropion.
    D. Oromandibular dystonia.

68. Methods of treating essential blepharospasm include all except:
    A. Surgical myectomy of affected areas.
    B. Chemical injection with doxorubicin.
    C. Oral benzodiazepines.
    D. Lid crutches.

69. Arterial occlusion following filler injection most commonly occur during the injection of :
    A. Upper eyelid
    B. Tear trough
    C. Glabella
    D. Crow's feet.

70. Reversal of filler injection can be done using :
    A. Deoxycholic acid
    B. Hyaluronidase
    C. Choline esterase
    D. Carbonic anhydrase.

71. In the lower lid, the medial fat pocket is separated from the middle fat pocket by the :
    A. Inferior rectus muscle
    B. Inferior oblique muscle
    C. Capsulopapebral fascia
    D. Lockwood ligament.

72. Deoxycholic acid injections in the lids results in :
    A. Flattening of wrinkling
    B. Reversal of filler action
    C. Dissolving fat pads
    D. Reversal of botulinum action.

Answers for this chapter Cosmetics and Injectables

1	C	19	D	37	D	55	D
2	D	20	A	38	B	56	A
3	C	21	D	39	B	57	B
4	D	22	D	40	D	58	A
5	D	23	D	41	D	59	A
6	D	24	A	42	B	60	C
7	D	25	D	43	C	61	D
8	B	26	D	44	A	62	A
9	C	27	D	45	A	63	A
10	C	28	C	46	C	64	A
11	C	29	B	47	B	65	B
12	C	30	D	48	D	66	C
13	C	31	A	49	B	67	C
14	B	32	D	50	C	68	D
15	B	33	D	51	A	69	C
16	A	34	C	52	A	70	B
17	A	35	D	53	B	71	B
18	B	36	D	54	A	72	C

The Lacrimal System

Nadeen El Toukhy

Tearing, a common complaint in the daily oculoplastic clinic can result from dry eyes, hypersecretion of tears, eyelids or eyelash malpositioning, or more commonly from stenosis or obstruction in the lacrimal drainage system. Disorders of the lacrimal drainage system, which cause tearing, discharge, or medial canthal swelling, are common ophthalmic complaints and account for about 3% of visits to general ophthalmology clinics. Accurate evaluation and localization of the pathology is essential for proper treatment and management.

Dry eyes disease is one of the most commonly encountered ocular surface diseases affecting millions of people. The severity varies over a wide spectrum and there are multiple diagnostic and treatment options available. Most of the cases are managed by conservative treatment. Newer treatment modalities help improve patient compliance.

Meibomian gland dysfunction (MGD) defined as a chronic, diffuse abnormality of the meibomian glands, is commonly characterized by terminal duct obstruction and/or qualitative/quantitative changes in the glandular secretion

Tests for dry eyes and MGD include Ocular surface disease index (OSDI), Schirmer's test, tear break-up time, tear osmolarity, Meibography, corneal and conjunctival staining with dyes as fluorescein.

Treatment of dry eyes include tear Supplementation, anti-inflammatory therapy, meibomian glands heat therapy, lacrimal occlusive devices and neurostimulation

Lacrimal Obstruction

Congenital nasolacrimal duct obstruction (CNLDO) is the most common ocular abnormality in children, aged less than 1year. Noncanalization of the inferior caudal end of the duct is the most common cause. Spontaneous resolution of the obstruction occurs in 96% of the children in the first year of life. Conservative management including lacrimal sac massage and antibiotics, is the mainstay in this age group. For older children nasolacrimal probing efficiently deals with most of the obstructions, however, the timing for probing remains controversial. The other invasive treatments like silicon tube intubation, balloon catheter dilation or dacryocystorhinostomy may be considered in cases refractory to probing.

Lacrimal punctal stenosis, despite being a common cause of epiphora, is frequently missed and often misdiagnosed. Moreover, available management guidelines are inconsistent and lack integrity. More understanding of the pathophysiology, etiology, clinical grading and diagnosis of this punctal disorder ie required.

N. El Toukhy (✉)
University of Pennsylvania, Philadelphia, USA
e-mail: nadineeltoukhy@yahoo.com

© The Author(s), under exclusive license to Springer Nature Switzerland AG 2021
E. A. El Toukhy (ed.), *Oculoplasty for Ophthalmologists*, https://doi.org/10.1007/978-3-030-68469-3_6

Chronic inflammation and subsequent fibrosis is the basic ultra-structure response to various noxious stimuli and appears to be the current proposed mechanism for acquired punctal stenosis. Longstanding treatment with several topical anti glaucoma agents, such as timolol, latanoprost, betaxolol and pilocarpine have been associated with punctal stenosis. Other topical agents have also been suggested as causes, and are often administered simultaneously. They include prednisolone acetate, dexamethasone, chloramphenicol, tobramycin, adrenaline, naphazoline, tropicamide, indomethacin, and mitomycin C. Punctal affection may be related to the medication themselves, the preservatives in the commercial preparations or the duration of treatment. The term "**Dacryotoxicity**" was introduced by the editor (ElToukhy) in 1999 to describe this effect. The use of these topical medications results in changes in the chemical and physical properties of the tears drained by the punctum (e.g. Ph, solutes' concentration, suspensions, ….) to which the delicate punctual epithelium reacts by inflammation and later fibrosis. Treatment includes the 3 snip procedure which is the most popular and has been advocated by many as the most successful treatment. Lacrimal stenting procedures can also be used.

Canalicular obstruction and stenosis can be either congenital or more commonly acquired. With inflammation, there is usually swelling in the area of the canaliculus, and the punctum is erythematous and raised (the so-called "pouting punctum" sign. Anatomically, the canalicular obstructions can be proximal canalicular (first 2-3 mm of canaliculus), mid canalicular (3-6 mm) or distal canalicular (beyond 6-8mm of normal canaliculus). Diagnosis can be easily made with syringing and a carefully done gentle probing which shows a typical 'soft' stop as the probe encounters soft tissue obstruction within the canaliculus, compared to a 'hard' stop seen in nasolacrimal duct obstructions. A thin probe, preferably not larger than 00 should be used gently and never forced inside the canaliculus to avoid creating a false passage. Treatment is difficult and includes: Canalicular Trephination,

Conjunctivodacryocystorhinostomy: Retrograde intubation dacryocystorhinostomy, or botulinum toxin injection into the lacrimal gland.

Acquired NLD obstruction is a relatively benign condition that can result from inflammation of unknown causes and eventually lead to secondary acquired stenosis and occlusive fibrosis of the lumen of the NLD. It is more common in elderly patients and affects women twice as frequently as men. It is most commonly an idiopathic involutional stenosis. Diagnosis can be easily reached by a combination of fluorescein dye disappearance test (DDT), lacrimal drainage system irrigation and diagnostic probing. Classically; in patients with acquired NLD obstruction, DCR is the treatment of choice. External DCR has a higher success rate than Endonasal DCR, can be done under local anesthesia, requires no expensive instrumentation, has a shorter learning curve, and when properly done, leaves no scar. Stenting may be used in certain patients with DCR.

Treatment of acute dacryocystitis includes pain relief, warm compresses, topical and systemic antibiotics. Once the acute dacryocystitis settles, most patients require a dacryocystorhinostomy (within 2–3 weeks) as a result of blockage within the nasolacrimal duct.

Lacrimal

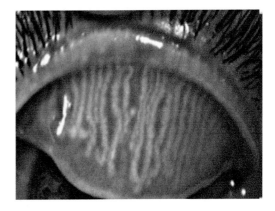

1. The above figure is :
   A. Flurophotometry
   B. Meibography
   C. Interferometry
   D. Meniscometry.

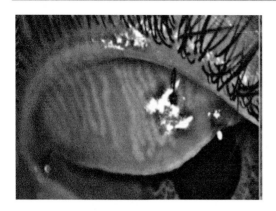

2. The above figure represent which grade of gland loss :
   A. Grade 0 : normal
   B. Grade 1 : <33%
   C. Grade 2 : <50%
   D. Grade 3 : >50%.

3. The nasolacrimal duct opens at the level of
   A. Spheno-ethmoidal recess
   B. Superior meatus
   C. Middle meatus
   D. Inferior meatus.

4. The anterior nasal opening (nares) leads to :
   A. Spheno-ethmoidal recess
   B. Superior meatus
   C. Middle meatus
   D. Inferior meatus.

5. The length of the lacrimal system in a 1 year old is ;
   A. 12–15 mm
   B. 18–20 mm
   C. 24–28 mm
   D. 28–32 mm.

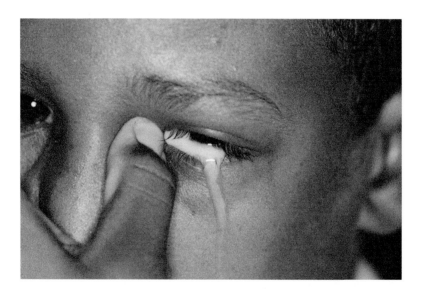

6. The above patient needs :
   A. Antibiotics
   B. Intubation
   C. DCR
   D. CDCR.

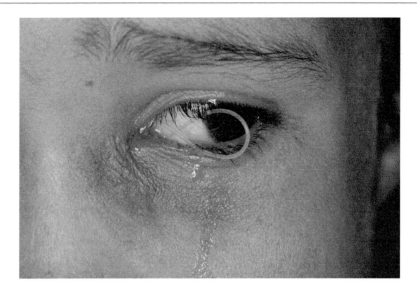

7. The above patient needs :
   A. Antibiotics
   B. Extubation
   C. Reinsertion of the tubes
   D. DCR.

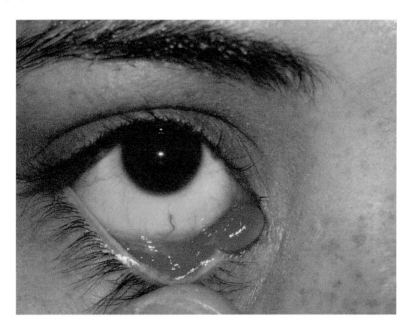

8. The above is a complication of :
   A. Canaliculitis
   B. NLD obstruction
   C. Silicone intubation
   D. Jones tube placement.

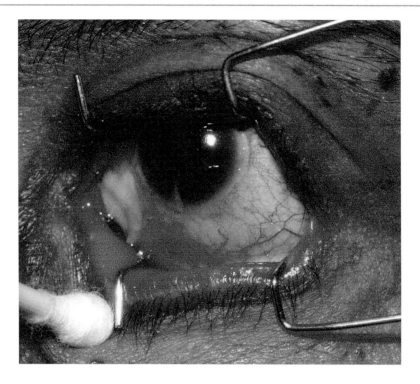

9. The above is a complication of :
   A. Canaliculitis
   B. NLD obstruction
   C. Silicone intubation
   D. Jones tube placement.

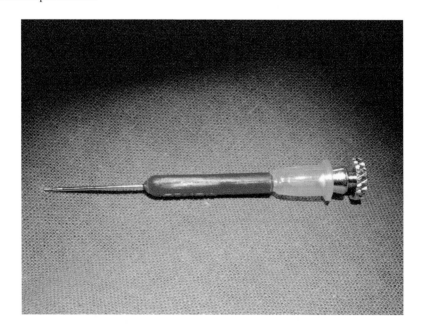

10. The above is a :
    A. Monocanalicular tube
    B. Mini Monoka
    C. Metereau tube
    D. Lacrimal trephine.

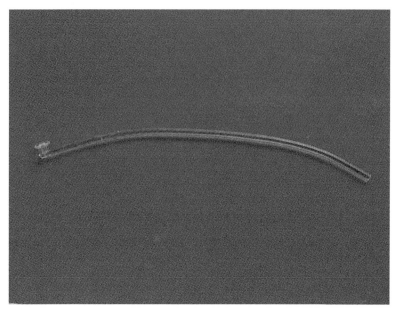

11. The above is a :
    A. Monocanalicular tube
    B. Mini Monoka
    C. Metereau tube
    D. Lacrimal trephine.

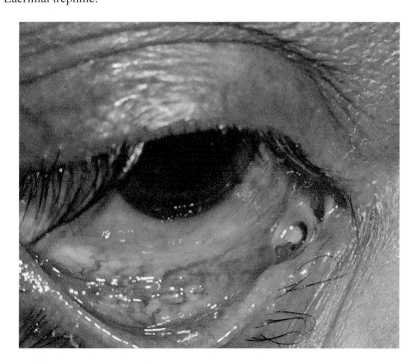

12. The above is a :
    A. Monocanalicular tube
    B. Mini Monoka
    C. Metereau tube
    D. Jones tube.

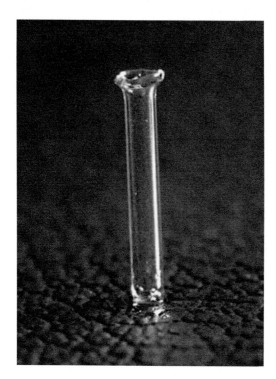

13. The above is a :
    A. Monocanalicular tube
    B. Mini Monoka
    C. Metereau tube
    D. Jones tube.

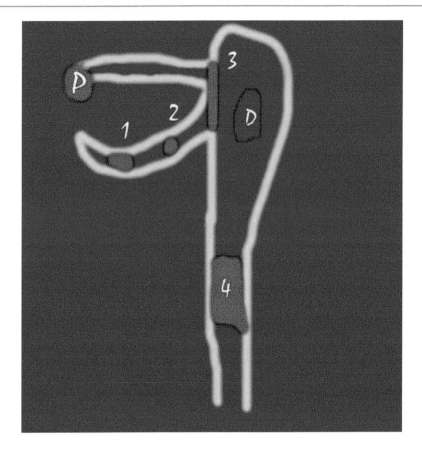

14. Obstruction at P requires :
   A. Plug
   B. Three snip procedure
   C. Intubation
   D. Dilatation.

15. Obstruction at 1 requires :
   A. Mini Monoka
   B. Three snip procedure
   C. Intubation
   D. Dilatation.

16. Obstruction at 2 requires :
   A. Lacrimal trephine
   B. Mini Monoka
   C. Intubation
   D. DCR.

17. Obstruction at 3 requires :
   a. DCR
   b. Lacrimal trephine
   c. Intubation
   d. Jones tube.

18. Obstruction at D requires :
   A. DCR
   B. Lacrimal trephine
   C. Intubation
   D. Jones tube Plug.

19. Obstruction at 4 requires
   A. DCR
   B. Lacrimal trephine
   C. Intubation
   D. Jones tube.

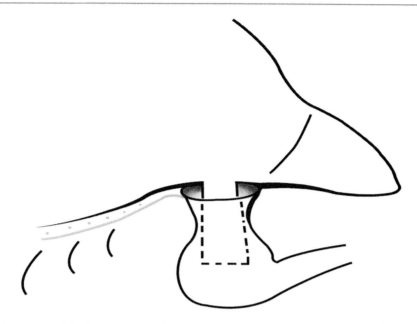

20. The above is used in the treatment of :
    A. Puntal obstruction
    B. Canalicular obstruction
    C. Pouting punctum
    D. Canaliculitis.

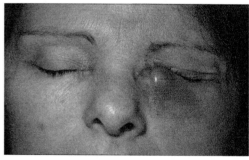

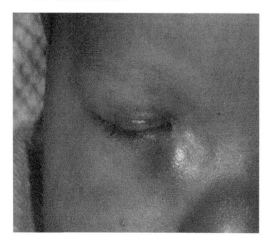

21. Treatment of this condition is ;
    A. Antibiotics
    B. Massage
    C. Probing
    D. Intubation.

22. Treatment of this condition is ;
    A. Antibiotics
    B. Incision
    C. Intubation
    D. DCR.

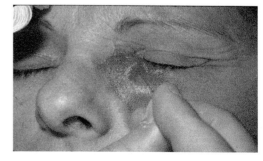

23. The above patient will develop
    A. Chronic dacyocystitis
    B. Lacrimal fistula
    C. Preseptal cellulitis
    D. Orbital cellulitis.

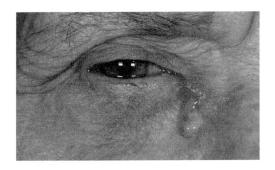

24. The Above patient has :
    A. Chronic dacyocystitis
    B. Lacrimal fistula
    C. Preseptal cellulitis
    D. Orbital cellulitis.

25. A 6 months old child present with history of epiphora and recent swelling over lacrimal sac area with discharge, the most appropriate management is:
    A. Treatment with topical antibiotics.
    B. Treatment with systemic antibiotics.
    C. Immediate probing
    D. Massaging and observation.

26. Osteotomy of which bone is done for making opening in DCR:
    A. Ethmoid
    B. Lacrimal
    C. Frontal process of maxilla
    D. Inferior meatus.

27. Regarding the canaliculi:
    A. Papillary conjunctivitis is present.
    B. Actinomyces Israeli is a frequently isolated pathogen.
    C. It is a self-limiting disease.
    D. Canaliculotomy when performed should involve both the horizontal and vertical canaliculi.

28. Regarding DCR, one of the following is an indication for surgery:
    A. Incomplete nasolacrimal duct obstruction.
    B. Persistence of epiphora.
    C. Resolved single episode of dacryocystitis.
    D. Painful distension of the lacrimal sac.

29. Regarding nasolacrimal canal one of the following statement is true:
    A. The nasolacrimal fossa is formed by maxillary and lacrimal bones.
    B. The bony nasolacrimal duct is located at the posterior medial wall.
    C. It empties into the middle meatus.
    D. Nasolacrimal duct (NLD) is 19mm in adults.

30. The most physiological test for assessment of lacrimal drainage system will be:
    A. Syringing
    B. Dacryocystography
    C. Lacrimal scintigraphy
    D. Jones II.

31. A 15-month-old girl presents with tearing and discharge from the left eye since birth. Which of the following is true regarding this condition?
    A. The condition is likely to resolve spontaneously
    B. The appropriate treatment is nasolacrimal duct probing
    C. Dye disappearance testing is likely to show no asymmetry
    D. Punctual abnormalities are likely to be the cause.

32. A 65-year-old man presents with tearing and discharge. On examination, irrigation of the lower canaliculus produces mucopurulent reflux. Which one of the following is true about this condition?
    A. Jones testing will reveal dye in the nose
    B. The condition is likely to resolve with a course of antibiotics
    C. There is probably a common canalicular block
    D. The correct treatment is dacryocystorhinostomy.

33. During dacryocystorhinostomy the osteotomy site is located in which one of the following locations?
    A. Is within 10 mm of the cribriform plate

B. Enlarges the opening of the common duct
C. Is adjacent to the valve of Hasner
D. Is adjacent to the superior turbinate.

34. A 50-year-old patient has a 2-day history of left-sided medial canthal swelling, pain, redness, and tearing. Few weeks before, he noted intermittent epiphora and swelling that could be relieved with digital massage. On examination, his visual acuity was 6/6 OU. Medial canthal and lower-eyelid edema and erythema were present. In regards to the treatment of this condition:
    A. Cool compresses are applied to the medial canthus
    B. Most adults will need a DCR for correction of outflow obstruction
    C. Topical antibiotics without systemic antibiotics should be prescribed
    D. Diagnostic probing may be therapeutic in adults.

35. A patient presenting with acute, severe pain in the medial canthal region with minimal enlargement of the lacrimal sac with no inflammation is most likely to have which of the following condition?
    A. Acute dacryocystitis
    B. Chronic dacryocystitis
    C. *Actinomyces* canaliculitis
    D. Impacted dacryolith.

36. With regards to congenital nasolacrimal duct obstruction :
    A. 50% resolve in the first year of life
    B. Imperforate membrane at the valve of Hasner is present in half of newborns

C. Long-term topical antibiotics have no rule in the management
D. Probing should be performed before the age of 6 months.

37. A newborn presented with swelling over the lacrimal sac , above the medial canthal tendon , the child has no breathing problem and there is no evidence of infection , the most appropriate next step is:
    A. Observation
    B. MRI to rule out meningoencephalcele
    C. Initiation of antibiotics
    D. Massaging of the sac.

38. A 65 years old woman complains of tearing and discharge. Irrigation of the lower canaliculus produces mucopurulent reflux from both puncti. All are true except;
    A. Jones testing will not reveal dye in the nose .
    B. There is probably a common canalicular block.
    C. Most likely diagnosis is lacrimal duct obstruction.
    D. Correct treatment is dacryocystorhinostomy.

39. A 5-month-old boy is presented with epiphora due to nasolacrimal duct obstruction. What is the preferred initial treatment?
    A. Digital massage
    B. Warm compresses
    C. Oral antibiotics
    D. Urgent surgery.

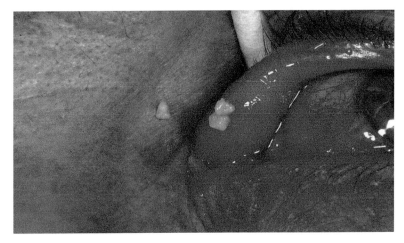

40. What is the most appropriate management option ?
    A. Aspiration of the mass with a large bore needle for biopsy
    B. Curettage with possible incision of punctum
    C. Dacryocystorhinostomy DCR
    D. Curettage and incision with irrigation of canaliculus with povidone iodine or fortified penicillin.

41. A 12 months old child has had tearing and discharge from the right eye since birth. Which of the following statements is true?
    A. Dye disappearance test is likely to show symmetry.
    B. This condition is likely to resolve spontaneously.
    C. The appropriate treatment is nasolacrimal duct probing.
    D. Punctual abnormalities are likely to be the cause.

42. Which gland does NOT contribute to the aqueous layer of the tear film?
    A. Krause.
    B. Main lacrimal
    C. Zeis.
    D. Wolfring.

43. What is the most common reason for failure of a DCR?
    A. Obstruction at the level of the common canaliculus or bony ostomy site.
    B. Unsuspected lacrimal sac tumor.

C. Recurrent infection of the lacrimal sac.
D. Dacryoliths (lacrimal stones).

44. Which one of the following is an indication for probing of the nasolacrimal system?
    A. Acute episode of acquired dacryocystitis.
    B. Intermittent acquired dacryocystitis.
    C. Congenital nasolacrimal duct obstruction unresponsive to massage.
    D. Work—up of all patients with epiphora.

45. In regard to canalicular trauma, all of the following are true EXCEPT:
    A. One may wait 24 to 48 hours after injury to allow soft tissue swelling to decrease.
    B. Upper canalicular trauma alone should never be surgically repaired so as not to risk damage to the remaining nasolacrimal system.
    C. Silicone stents should be left in place for 3 to 6 months.
    D. Surgical microanastomosis of the cut canalicular ends with silicone stent intubation offers the best possibility of successful repair.

46. Chronic use of the following medications has been reported to cause canalicular stenosis EXCEPT:
    A. Echothiophate.
    B. Idoxuridine.
    C. Epinephrine.
    D. Atropine.

47. The parasympathetic nerve fibers to the lacrimal gland travel through the following nerves EXCEPT:
    A. Deep petrosal nerve
    B. Greater petrosal nerve
    C. Zygomatic branch of the maxillary nerve
    D. Zygomaticotemporal nerve.

48. The following are true about the lacrimal gland EXCEPT:
    A. Receives its blood supply chiefly from a branch of the ophthalmic artery
    B. Contains capsule derived from the orbital septum
    C. Is divided into two lobes by the lateral horn of the levator aponeurosis
    D. Receives sensory supply from the trigeminal nerve.

49. The following are true about the nasolacrimal system, EXCEPT:
    A. The canaliculi are found within the medial canthus along their full lengths
    B. The lower canaliculus is longer than the upper canaliculus
    C. The canaliculus can be dilated to three times its size without affecting its integrity
    D. Sinus of Maier is found in the common canaliculus.

50. The following forms the lacrimal sac fossa:
    A. Lacrimal bone and orbital plate of maxilla.
    B. Lacrimal bone and ethmoid bone.
    C. Lacrimal bone and frontal process of maxilla.
    D. Lacrimal bone and nasal bone.

51. A 50 year old woman presented with an enlarging, tender, red mass in the right medial canthal area for 2 weeks. She has no history of facial trauma or surgery, but had a similar episode of medial canthal swelling and pain 8 months earlier that resolved with oral antibiotics and warm compresses. Examination revealed a mass in the right lower medial canthus with surrounding erythema and an elevated tear lake with mucoid debris. The puncti appeared normal in both eyes. What should be done for further management of this case?
    A. Urgent DCR
    B. DCR after a 2 week course of antibiotics
    C. Lacrimal probing and intubation
    D. Oral Antibiotics and warm compresses.

52. Which of the following is the treatment of canaliculitis?
    A.. Probing.
    B. Syringing.
    C. Dilatation.
    D. Canaliculotomy.

53. Mucin layer deficiency of tear film is seen in:
    A. Keratoconjunctivitis sicca
    B. Lacrimal gland removal
    C. Canalicular block
    D. Herpes zoster.

54. Epiphora means:
    A. Cerebrospinal fluid running from nose after fracture of anterior cranial fossa
    B. A presenting feature of a cerebral tumour
    C. An abnormal flow of tears due to obstruction of the lacrimal duct
    D. Eversion of lower eyelid following injury.

55. A 2 month-old child presents with epiphora and regurgitation of mucopurulent material: The likely diagnosis is:
    A. Mucopurulent conjunctivitis
    B. Congenital dacryocystitis
    C. Buphthalmos
    D. Encysted mucocoele.

56. Most common site of obstruction in congenital NLD obstruction:
    A. Upper canaliculus
    B. Lower canaliculus
    C. Common canaliculus
    D. Valve of Hasner.

57. Initial treatment of congenital dacryocystitis is:
    A. Massage
    B. Probing
    C. DCR
    D. Antibiotics.

58. Treatment of chronic dacryocystitis is:
    A. Dacryocystorhinostomy
    B. Antibiotics
    C. Probing
    D. Massage.

59. A 65-year-old woman presents with watering from her left eye since 2 years. Syringing revealed a patent drainage system. Rest of the examination was normal. A diagnosis of lacrimal pump failure was made. Confirmation of diagnosis is done by:
    A. Dacryoscintigraphy
    B. Dacryocystography
    C. Pressure syringing
    D. Canaliculus irrigation test.

60. Phenol red test for dry eye: True statement is:
    A. It requires topical anaesthesia
    B. It measures the volume of tears as it changes colour on contact with tears
    C. If colour changes to blue, it depicts mucin deficiency
    D. It requires a pH meter.

61. Distention of the lacrimal sac superior to the medial canthal tendon occurs in?
    A. Primary acquired nasolacrimal duct obstruction
    B. Canaliculitis
    C. Lacrimal sac tumor
    D. Dacryolithiasis.

62. As the bony nasolacrimal canal runs inferiorly it initially curves
    A. Medial and anterior
    B. Medial and posterior
    C. Lateral and anterior
    D. Lateral and posterior.

63. What percentage of infants are born with an imperforate valve of Hasner?
    A. 10%
    B. 20%
    C. 50%
    D. 80%.

64. Approximately how many days after birth do infants gain full tear production?
    A. 14 days
    B. 21 days
    C. 35 days
    D. 42 days.

65. The most common neoplasm of the lacrimal gland is the
    A. Adenoid cystic carcinoma
    B. Mucoepidermoid carcinoma
    C. Benign mixed tumor
    D. Adenocarcinoma.

66. The most common malignant neoplasm of the lacrimal gland is the
    A. Adenoid cystic carcinoma
    B. Mucoepidermoid carcinoma
    C. Maligant mixed tumor
    D. Adenocarcinoma.

67. What anatomic structure divides the lacrimal gland anteriorly into orbital and palpebral lobes?
    A. Orbital septum
    B. Periorbita
    C. Superior transverse ligament
    D. Levator aponeurosis.

68. A 40-year-old man presents with a one year history of gradually progressive painless proptosis of the right eye. CT reveals globular enlargement of the lacrimal gland with no extension anterior to the orbital rim. All of the following are true, except
    A. Initial approach to the patient should include an incisional biopsy
    B. Histopathology will show the tumor has a pseudocapsule
    C. Definitive treatment will necessitate lateral orbitotomy
    D. The most likely diagnosis is more frequently encountered in men.

69. In evaluating a child with tearing, all of the following are causes of reflex hypersecretion, except
    A. TORCH infection
    B. Congenital glaucoma
    C. Distichiasis
    D. Epiblepharon.

70. The average distance from the lacrimal punctum to the nasolacrimal sac is
    A. 2 mm
    B. 6 mm
    C. 10 mm
    D. 12 mm.

71. What is the organism that most commonly causes canaliculitis?
    A. Nocardia asteroides
    B. Staphylococcus
    C. Candida a/bicans
    D. Actinomyces israelii.

72. All of the following medications are known to potentially cause canalicular obstruction, except
    A. Phospholine iodine
    B. 5-fluorouracil
    C. Doxorubicin
    D. Idoxuridine.

73. What type of epithelium are the lacrimal canaliculi lined by?
    A. Stratified cuboidal
    B. Pseudostratified ciliated columnar
    C. Stratified squamous
    D. Bilayered cuboidal.

74. An infant with congenital nasolacrimal duct obstruction undergoes lacrimal probing. Starting from the punctum, what distance will the probe travel before reaching the inferior meatus?
    A. 12 mm
    B. 20 mm
    C. 24 mm
    D. 30 mm.

75. In adults, the average distance from lacrimal punctum to inferior nasal meatus is
    A. 12 mm
    B. 18 mm
    C. 25 mm
    D. 30 mm.

76. What is the most commonly performed clinical test in the evaluation of the adult patient with epiphora?
    A. Jones I test
    B. Jones II test
    C. Lacrimal irrigation
    D. Dye disappearance test.

77. Which one of the following functional tests of lacrimal drainage is most likely to yield a false-positive result?
    A. Lacrimal scintigraphy
    B. Secondary dye test (Jones II test)
    C. Dye disappearance test
    D. Primary dye test (Jones I test).

78. Which one of the following functional tests of lacrimal drainage allows identification of a failure of the lacrimal pump mechanism?
    A. Schirmer's test
    B. Primary dye test (Jones I test)
    C. Dye disappearance test
    D. Secondary dye test (Jones II test).

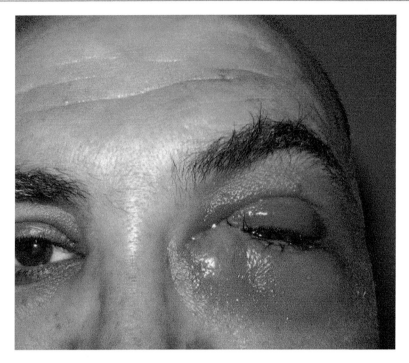

79. Which is the most appropriate initial step in the treatment of this patient?
    A. Dacryocystorhinostomy
    B. Broad-spectrum antibiotics
    C. Nasolacrimal duct probing
    D. Canalicular irrigation.

80. The most important predisposing factor for acute dacryocystitis is
    A. Chronic blepharitis
    B. Acute bacterial conjunctivitis
    C. Dry eye
    D. Tear stasis.

81. When performing an endoscopic dacryo-cyst-rhinostomy, part of the following bones are often removed, except
    A. Nasal
    B. Maxilla
    C. Lacrimal
    D. Ethmoid.

82. Acute, lancinating pain in the medial canthal region with minimal noninflamed enlargement of the lacrimal sac is most suggestive of
    A. Impacted dacryolith
    B. Acute dacryocystitis

C. Chronic dacryocystitis
D. Wegener granulomatosis.

83. The most common site of organic obstruction in acquired nasolacrimal obstruction is
    A. Punctum
    B. Canaliculus
    C. Intraosseous nasolacrimal duct
    D. Valve of Hasner.

84. All of the following conditions may present with epiphora secondary to impaired blink function except
    A. Sjogren's syndrome
    B. Parkinson's disease
    C. Scleroderma
    D. Progressive supranuclear palsy.

85. Which of the following glands are matched with their correct types of secretions?
    A. Moll-apocrine, main lacrimal gland-eccrine, meibomian glands-apocrine
    B. Glands of Krause-holocrine, gland of Zeis-apocrine, goblet cells-holocrine
    C. Glands of Wolfring-eccrine, gland of Moll-apocrine, goblet cells-holocrine
    D. Main lacrimal gland-eccrine, meibomian glands-holocrine, gland of Zeis-apocrine.

86. The (OSDI) is used to diagnose:
    A. Severity of epiphora
    B. Severity of dry eyes
    C. Level of lacrimal obstruction
    D. Sjogren syndrome.

87. All of the following statements are true in describing the lacrimal gland *except:*
    A. The lateral horn of the levator separates the orbital and palpebral lobes
    B. The orbital and palpebral lobes have separate excretory glands that empty into the conjunctival fornix approximately 5 mm above the superior margin of the tarsus
    C. The lacrimal glands are exocrine glands
    D. Blood supply is provided by the lacrimal artery, a branch of the ophthalmic artery

88. The osteotomy site fashioned at the time of a dacryocystorhinostomy (DCR):
    A. Is adjacent to the valve of Hasner
    B. Enlarges the opening of the common duct
    C. Is adjacent to the superior turbinate
    D. Is within 10 mm of the cribriform plate.

89. The Jones I test (primary dye test):
    A. Accurately defines the location of a nasolacrimal system obstruction
    B. Involves irrigating the lacrimal sac with fluid
    C. Has a high false-negative rate
    D. Is a reliable indicator of nasolacrimal duct obstruction.

90. What is the most frequently seen primary malignant tumor of the lacrimal sac?
    A. Fibrous histiocytoma
    B. Hemangiopericytoma
    C. Squamous cell carcinoma
    D. Lymphoma.

91. Which one of the following is an indication for probing of the nasolacrimal system?
    A. Acute episode of acquired dacryocystitis
    B. Intermittent acquired inflammatory nasolacrimal system obstruction
    C. Congenital nasolacrimal duct obstruction unresponsive to massage
    D. Workup of all patients with epiphora.

92. Adult patients presenting with epiphora with a complete obstruction at the sac-duct junction would be expected to have:
    A. Negative dye disappearance test/positive Jones III
    B. Positive dye disappearance test/positive Jones I
    C. Positive dye disappearance test/negative Jones I
    D. Negative dye disappearance test/negative Jones II.

93. Which one of the following statements regarding dacryocystograms is *true?*
    A. They are a required part of the workup in acquired nasolacrimal system obstruction
    B. They are an excellent test for nasolacrimal function
    C. They demonstrate canaliculi well
    D. They demonstrate the nasolacrimal sac well.

94. All of the following statements regarding tumors of the nasolacrimal sac are true *except:*
    A. They may produce painless irreducible swelling of the lacrimal sac
    B. They may produce bleeding on attempted probing
    C. They do not usually produce secondary dacryocystitis
    D. They may produce epiphora.

95. Regarding the canalicular system, which statement is *false?*
    A. The ampulla has the largest diameter of the canalicular system
    B. A common canaliculus is present in approximately 30% of the population
    C. The canaliculus has a diameter of approximately 1.0 mm
    D. The average distance from the punctum to the nasolacrimal sac is approximately 10 mm.

96. Regarding irrigation of lacrimal outflow system, which statement is *false?*
    A. Syringing saline into the lower canaliculus that irrigates into the nose indicates that no obstruction exists and that the system is functioning normally
    B. Irrigation of the upper punctum with regurgitation through the upper punctum suggests an upper canalicular obstruction
    C. Irrigation of the lower canaliculus into the sac with complete regurgitation through the upper punctum suggests obstruction of the nasolacrimal sac or duct
    D. It may be helpful to recover fluid from the nose to examine for casts

97. All of the following are indications for a conjunctivodacryocystorhinostomy or CDCR (Jones tube procedure) *except:*
    A. Lacrimal canaliculi have been destroyed
    B. Canalicular remnants cannot be anastomosed with the intranasal cavity
    C. Common canalicular obstruction combined with nasolacrimal duct obstruction
    D. Paralytic or scarred eyelids with absent canalicular pumping mechanism.

98. In acute dacryocystitis:
    A. Topical antibiotics without systemic antibiotics should be prescribed
    B. Cold compresses are applied to the medial canthus
    C. Diagnostic probing may be therapeutic in adults
    D. Most adults will need a DCR for correction of outflow obstruction.
    A 10-year-old boy involved in an accident few months ago has left-sided epiphora since the accident, along with a 1-week history of fever and progressive swelling, redness, and pain in the left medial canthal region with mucopurulent discharge from the medial canthus:

99. Appropriate initial workup of this patient includes all of the following *except:*
    A. A complete ophthalmic exam
    B. CT scan of the orbits and sinuses
    C. Probing and irrigation of the left nasolacrimal system
    D. Culture and Gram stain of the medial canthal discharge.

100. Appropriate initial therapy of this patient would include all of the following *except:*
    A. DCR
    B. IV antibiotics
    C. Topical antibiotic drops
    D. Incision and drainage of any pointing abscess.

101. In acquired nasolacrimal system obstruction, where is the blockage most frequently located?
    A. Canaliculi
    B. Nasolacrimal sac
    C. Nasolacrimal duct
    D. Inferior turbinate.

102. What is the most common bacterial etiology in acute dacryocystitis?
    A. Actinomyces israelii
    B. Pseudomonas aeruginosa
    C. Streptococcus pneumoniae
    D. Staphylococcal species.
    A 12-month-old child has right-sided epiphora since birth. The mother has been massaging the right nasolacrimal sac for the past 6 months with no improvement:

103. In congenital nasolacrimal system obstruction, where is the level of the obstruction?
    A. Common canaliculus
    B. Lacrimal sac
    C. Valve of Rosenmiiller
    D. Valve of Hasner.

104. The next therapeutic recommendation would include:
    A. Continuing massage
    B. Nasolacrimal system probing
    C. DCR

D. Cbservation, as most congenital obstructions resolve without therapy.

105. Silicone stent intubation (with possible inferior turbinate infracture) is indicated in this patient when:
    A. Massage therapy has proven unsuccessful
    B. Dacryocystography (DCG) shows obstruction at the level of the nasolacrimal duct
    C. Nasolacrimal system probing has proven unsuccessful
    D. The patient is older than 12 months.

The shown patient reports a 3-month history of intermittent tearing and mattering in her right medial canthus. Additionally, she has noted focal swelling and tenderness near her lid margins.

106. All of the following organisms are associated with canaliculitis *except:*
    A. Actinomyces
    B. Candida
    C. Acanthamoeba
    D. Streptomyces.

107. Which one of the following suggests a diagnosis of canaliculitis?
    A. Mucopurulent reflux from punctum with compression of the lacrimal sac
    B. Gritty sensation on probing with yellow-tinged concretions
    C. A palpable subcutaneous mass above the medial canthal tendon
    D. Palpable masses in the lacrimal sac.

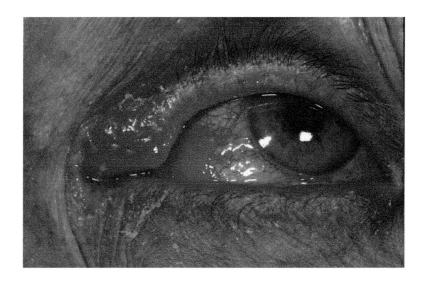

108. Treatment of canaliculitis includes all of the following *except:*
    A. Canalicular curettage
    B. Canalicular incision and debridement
    C. Canalicular irrigation
    D. DCR.

109. Adenoid cystic carcinoma of the lacrimal gland is best treated by:
    A. Exenteration and removal of involved bone
    B. Radiation therapy
    C. Chemotherapy
    D. All of the above.

110. What is the most common organism implicated in dacryocystitis?
    A. Non-septate fungi
    B. Gram-positive bacteria
    C. Septate fungi
    D. Gram-negative bacteria.

111. Blood-tinged tears should prompt what treatment?
    A. Balloon dacryoplasty
    B. Biopsy of lacrimal sac
    C. Probing and tube placement
    D. Dacryocystorhinostomy.

112. A patient with acute dacryocystitis, reflux of pus from the canaliculi, and preseptal cellulitis should be treated with which of the following?
    A. Immediate dacryocystorhinostomy
    B. Massage
    C. Systemic antibiotics
    D. Probing and irrigation for diagnosis confirmation.

113. What is the appropriate treatment for acute dacryocystitis with localized abscess?
    A. Irrigation and probing of the lacrimal sytem followed by application of warm compresses
    B. Oral antibiotics and drainage of abscess or immediate dacryocystorhinostomy
    C. Topical antibiotics
    D. Surgical creation of a permanent dacryocutaneous fistula.

114. What would be the preferred management to treat a patient with membranous, congenital, nasolacrimal duct obstruction and stenosis of both upper and lower canaliculi?
    A. Bicanalicular intubation of the nasolacrimal duct
    B. Bicanalicular intubation with dacrocystorhinostomy
    C. Monocanalicular intubation
    D. Bicanalicular ring intubation with pigtail probe.

115. When copious mucous refluxes from the superior canaliculus while irrigating through the inferior canaliculus, what is the most likely site of obstruction?
    A. Inferior canaliculus
    B. Superior canaliculus
    C. Nasolacrimal duct
    D. Common internal punctum.

116. A 1-week-old infant is having difficulty breathing due to bilateral congenital dacryocystocele. What management is needed?
    A. Urgent decompression in the operating room
    B. Systemic antibiotics
    C. Topical antibiotics and massage
    D. Bedside probing of the nasolacrimal duct.

117. Regarding dacryocystography, which is incorrect:
    A. Can define the site of complete lacrimal system obstruction
    B. Can visualize a filling defect in patients who have lacrimal sac tumo
    C. May evaluate lacrimal system physiologic function
    D. Can image compression or deflection of the lacrimal sac or duct.

118. Regarding congenital nasolacrimal obstruction, which is incorrect :
    A. Should usually be treated by about age 1 year with irrigation and probing
    B. Should be treated with silicone intubation after two failed probing attempts
    C. Associated with amnioceles requires probing at an early age
    D. Spontaneously resolves in more than 90% of patients by age 1 year.

119. Regarding dacryocystorhinostomy, which is incorrect:
    A. Has a success rate of 90%
    B. Requires a skin incision below the medial canthal tendon

C. May require incision of the anterior limb of the medial canthal tendon

D. Usually requires silicone tube placement.

120. A normal OSDI is :
A. Below 12
B. 13-22
C. 23-32
D. Above 33.

121. An increase of tear osmolarity above which value is seen in dry eyes?:
A. 290 mOsm/L
B. 300 mOsm/L
C. 310 mOsm/L
D. 320 mOsm/L.

122. An inflammatory component of dry eyes is confirmed by detection of which substance in tears :
A. Lysozyme
B. Lactoferrin
C. MMP-9
D. Cytokine.

123. Meibomian glands heat therapy entails temperatures of :
A. 40 C
B. 42 C
C. 44 C
D. 46 C.

124. Neurostimulation is used in treating :
A. MGD
B. Aqueous deficient dry eyes
C. Corneal epithelial defects
D. Goblet cell deficiency.

125. Dacrotoxicity entails :
A. Lacrimal obstruction caused by alkali injury
B. Lacrimal obstruction caused by eye drops
C. Lacrimal obstruction caused by trachoma
D. Lacrimal obstruction caused by iatrogenic injuries.

126. Punctal plugs are used in the management of all except:
A. Dry eyes
B. Punctal occlusion
C. Glaucoma patients on chronic medications
D. Post LASIK as a temporary measure.

Answers for this chapter Lacrimal System

1	B	33	A	65	C	97	C
2	C	34	B	66	A	98	D
3	D	35	D	67	D	99	C
4	C	36	B	68	A	100	A
5	B	37	B	69	A	101	C
6	C	38	B	70	C	102	C
7	B	39	A	71	D	103	D
8	C	40	D	72	C	104	B
9	D	41	C	73	C	105	C
10	D	42	C	74	B	106	C
11	B	43	A	75	D	107	B
12	D	44	C	76	C	108	D
13	D	45	A	77	D	109	D
14	B	46	D	78	D	110	B
15	A	47	A	79	B	111	B
16	A	48	B	80	D	112	C
17	A	49	A	81	A	113	D
18	A	50	C	82	A	114	A
19	A	51	B	83	C	115	C
20	A	52	D	84	A	116	A
21	B	53	D	85	C	117	C
22	B	54	C	86	B	118	C
23	B	55	B	87	B	119	D
24	B	56	D	88	D	120	A
25	B	57	A	89	C	121	C
26	C	58	A	90	C	122	C
27	B	59	A	91	C	123	B
28	C	60	B	92	C	124	B
29	A	61	C	93	D	125	B
30	C	62	D	94	C	126	C
31	B	63	C	95	B		
32	D	64	D	96	A		

Trauma

Essam A. El Toukhy

Eyelid, adnexal and orbital injuries can be a part of multisystem trauma. The basic ABCs of the trauma management should be considered and applied in every trauma patient. This includes securing a patent airway and stabilization of the circulation. Ophthalmic evaluation and management are deferred until more serious problems are addressed.

Once the patient is stable, attention could be directed to the eye and orbital injuries. The patient should be evaluated for any globe or optic nerve injuries. This may be difficult especially in patients who are unconscious or uncooperative. The eyelid may be swollen and difficult to open, so care should be taken to avoid forceful opening of the eyelid as this may worsen the already traumatized globe.

Circumstances of the injury can help determine the type and extent of the trauma. The mechanism of injury can give an idea about the depth of the wound as well as the possibility of foreign body presence.

This should include evaluation of the globe, adnexal tissue, orbit and face. If the patient is conscious and cooperative, visual acuity, pupillary responses, intraocular pressure measurement as well as dilated fundus examination should be performed. Sometimes examination under anesthesia can be done to avoid further globe injuries during manipulation of the eyelid.

The eyelid is examined for the extent of the wound and if it involves the septum, the muscle, lid margin or canaliculus. Canalicular injury is suspected when the injury lies medial to the punctum. Medial or lateral canthal injuries as well as tissue loss should be ruled out

Most lid wounds could be repaired under local anesthesia using lidocaine1% with epinephrine 1:100,000. This can be done in the emergency room if minor or in the operative theatre in most injuries. General anesthesia is reserved for extensive injuries, associated canalicular injuries or poorly cooperative patients. Nerve blocks are ideal in such situations.

It should be remembered to reestablish the integrity of the basic lid parts; anterior lamella, posterior lamella, the lid retractors mainly the levator, the canaliculi and the canthal tendons.

Tissue loss may be in anterior lamella or it can be full thickness involving the lid margin. In such conditions, it should be remembered to avoid undue tension on the wound margins. This situation can be dealt with in a manner similar to lid reconstruction after tumor excision.

Canalicular lesions may be missed. They should be suspected in injuries medial to the punctum that may be laterally displaced. The diagnosis is confirmed by direct visualization of the cut edge or passing a probe into the canaliculus.

E. A. El Toukhy (✉)
Oculoplasty Service, Cairo University, Cairo, Egypt
e-mail: eeltoukhy@yahoo.com

Early repair of the canalicular injury is much easier and more successful than late repair or conjunctivo dacryocystorhinostomy with Jones tube. This must be done under the microscope with high magnification. It can also be identified using injection of a fluorescein dye or vesicoelastic material or air. A stent should be placed through the transected canaliculus. Bicanalicular silicone tube is commonly used however, some surgeons use monocanalicular tubes. Destruction of the upper lacrimal system especially with chemical injuries and obliteration of the canaliculi usually necessitates conjunctiveodacryocystorhinostomy (CDCR) with insertion of Lister Jones tube. Chronic dacryocystitis or complete NLD obstruction are treated by conventional DCR.

Lacrimal passage injuries associated with orbital or nasal fractures may be overlooked especially with the edema or ecchymosis. However, associated nasal bone fractures as well as traumatic telecanthus should raise the index of suspicion.

A nasoethmoidal fracture usually results from a force delivered across the nasal bridge and it is very common in automobile accidents in which the face strikes the dashboard. The nasal bones become fractured and displaced. The lacrimal and sphenoidal bones are usually crushed. They are associated with surgical emphysema. Traumatic telecanthus is usually present in association with lacrimal passage injury.

Wounds of the eye brow should be meticulously sutured with proper alignment of the upper and lower border of the brows. If the wound is deep it should be closed in layers to minimize scar stretching. However many wounds of the eye brow will show few weeks after healing as a hairless scar. This could be managed by scar revision and follicular hair transplantation from the opposite or the same brow.

Evaluation of the orbit includes searching for ocular motility deficit, surgical emphysema, hyposthesia of the check, nose or upper lip in addition to palpable orbital rim fractures. Orbital imaging with CT is requested when orbital wall fracture or presence of foreign body is suspected.

A significant orbital trauma can result in a range of manifestations from orbital contusion to an orbital wall fracture. Orbital wall fractures may also less commonly occur with a penetrating injury. Whenever a penetrating orbital injury is present, the patient must be evaluated for the presence of an intraorbital foreign body.

Although most orbital injuries are self-limiting, orbital trauma may result in serious sequelae that may require emergent intervention such as orbital hemorrhage, traumatic optic neuropathy and oculocardiac reflex secondary to an impinged rectus muscle.

Orbital fractures usually present in the setting of a blunt trauma to the orbit and face. The term orbital blow out fracture implies increase in the orbital volume secondary to an outward deformity in the inferior and/or medial orbital wall(s) which occurs following an impact to the orbit by an object that is equal to or larger than the dimensions of the orbital aperture. This deformity may be accompanied by herniation of the orbital contents into the adjacent cavities; namely the maxillary or ethmoid paranasal sinuses.

The infraorbital groove, which is located medially in the floor, is an area of weakness, thus orbital floor fractures are usually located in its vicinity. This is an important landmark in relation to orbital floor fractures as damage to the infraorbital nerve presents with loss of sensation in the cheek, side of nose and upper lip. The floor of the orbit is the roof of the underlying maxillary sinus.

Nausea, vomiting, palpitations and sweating may be symptoms of oculocardiac reflex secondary to entrapment of an extraocular muscle, which more commonly occurs in children.

Orbital floor fractures in children tend to differ from those in adults. This is due to the elastic nature of bones in children, which result in greenstick fractures and 'trap-door' phenomenon. Similarly the Oculocardiac reflex and the white-eyed blow out fractures are conditions that are seen in mostly only children.

The preferred imaging technique is computerized tomography (CT) without intravenous contrast. This is the most sensitive imaging technique delineating orbital wall fractures. It outlines the location, extent and comminution of fractures, as well as the presence of extraocular muscles and orbital soft tissue entrapment.

In children with extraocular muscle impingement, release of the impinged muscle and orbital wall fracture repair should be performed within 24 to 48 hours of the injury. Patients with oculocardiac reflex must be operated immediately. Repairing fractures in the first 8 days after trauma has a better long term prognosis as regards motility and enophthalmos than repairing after 8 days.

Orbital floor fractures can be approached transcutaneously through a subciliary or lower eyelid crease incision. However, transconjunctival approach through the inferior tarsal conjunctiva is preferred for better cosmetic outcome. The fracture is identified, prolapsed tissues are restored back and an implant material is fashioned to cover the defect completely and overlapping the surrounding intact bone by 3–4 mm circumferentially.

Trauma to the orbit can also result in other types of injuries including: orbital roof fractures, mid-facial fractures, traumatic orbital hemorrhage, surgical emphysema, carotid cavernous fistula or septic cavernous sinus thrombosis.

Trauma

1. The lacrimal drainage system is usually injured in which type of Le Forte fractures?
   A. Le Forte I
   B. Le Forte II
   C. Le Forte III
   D. All 3 types.
2. Numbness due to an orbital blowout fracture is due to:
   A. Entrapment of the infraorbital nerve distal to the foramen
   B. Fracture of the body of the zygoma
   C. Fracture of the infraorbital rim
   D. Injury of the infraorbital nerve within the orbital floor.

3. Typical finding of blowout fracture of the orbital, one is false:
   A. Ecchymosis and edema of the eyelids
   B. Diplopia
   C. Exophthalmos
   D. Emphysema of the orbit and eyelids.
4. The most serious danger to vision is:
   A. A blow to the eye ball
   B. Fracture through sphenoid bone
   C. Monocular proptosis
   D. Orbital cellulitis.
5. The most common organism in trauma-associated preseptal cellulitis is:
   A. Haemophilus influenzae
   B. Streptococcus pneumoniae
   C. Bacillus cereus
   D. Staphylococcus aureus.
6. A man presented with injury of the left brow with a stick. visual acuity is 20/20 OD and 20/200 OS. Examination revealed proptosis of the left eye with a large tense eyelid hematoma and subconjunctival hemorrhage. Pupils showed left RAPD. Fundus showed pulsating central retinal artery of the left eye. What would be the most appropriate immediate management?
   A. Paracentesis
   B. Begin intravenous corticosteroids
   C. Intravenous mannitol 20%
   D. Lateral canthotomy and cantholysis.
7. The most likely pathophysiology for diplopia development in the setting of traumatic carotid cavernous fistula is:
   A. Damage to the third cranial nerve from elevated intracranial pressure
   B. Compression of the sixth cranial nerve within the cavernous sinus
   C. Compression of the fourth cranial nerve
   D. Disturbed eye movements due to orbital edema.
8. Which of the following findings is Not associated with orbital floor fractures?
   A. Late enophthalmos few weeks after the fracture
   B. Tear drop sign on CT scan
   C. Unilateral mid-facial sensory loss
   D. Rapid improvement in traumatic diplopia over a 24-hour period.

9. First choice in the evaluation of acute orbital trauma is:
   A. Orbital ultrasound
   B. Palpation
   C. CT scan
   D. MRI.

10. Indications for repair of orbital blow out fracture include all of the following except;
    A. Fracture involving more than half of the orbital floor
    B. Inferior rectus weakness
    C. Pain and oculocardiac reflex on upgaze
    D. Significant inferior rectus entrapment.

11. A patient is struck on the right eye. Radiography shows a fracture of the right orbital floor, forced duction test cannot be done due to poor cooperation. 2 days after the injury, 3 mm of right exophthalmos is present, movement of the eye is restricted in up gaze, down gaze and horizontal gaze. Treatment should be;
    A. Urgent lateral canthotomy
    B. Caldwell–luc incision and packing of the maxillary sinus
    C. Skin incision over the inferior orbital rim and covering the fracture defect with a plastic plate
    D. Skin incision beneath the eye lash and covering of the fracture defect with a plastic plate.

12. In regard to canalicular trauma, all of the following are true EXCEPT:
    A. One may wait 24 to 48 hours after injury to allow soft tissue swelling to decrease
    B. Upper canalicular trauma alone should never be surgically repaired so as not to risk damage to the remaining nasolacrimal system
    C. Silicone stents should be left in place for 3 to 6 months
    D. Surgical microanastomosis of the cut canalicular ends with silicone stent intubation offers the best possibility of successful repair.

13. Where do orbital floor fractures most commonly occur?
    A. Along the infraorbital canal

B. Within the zygoma medial to the infra-robital canal
C. Within the zygoma medial to the infra-robital fissure
D. Within the maxilla medial to the infra-robital canal.

14. In exploring upper eyelid trauma with a full-thickness laceration involving the eyelid margin, the physician must be aware of the order in which the anatomical structures are normally encountered. The correct order is:
    A. Skin, orbicularis muscle, preaponeurotic fat, Muller's muscle, levator aponeurosis, conjunctiva
    B. Skin, preaponeurotic Fat, orbicularis muscle, septum, levator aponeurosis, Muller's muscle, conjunctiva
    C. Skin, orbicularis muscle, septum, preaponeurotic fat, levator aponeurosis Muller's muscle, conjunctiva
    D. Skin, orbicularis muscle, preaponeurotic fat, septum, levator aponeurosis, Muller's muscle, conjunctiva.

15. The most common site of blow out fracture is:
    A. Floor
    B. Lateral wall
    C. Medial wall
    D. Roof.

16. Blow out fracture of the orbit involves:
    A. Superior wall
    B. Postero-medial part of the orbital floor
    C. Medial wall
    D. Lateral wall.

17. True about blow out fracture of the orbit are except:
    A. Herniates into maxillary antrum
    B. Extraocular movements are restricted
    C. Looking down is easy
    D. Orbital floor reconstruction is the treatment.

18. Most common cause of fracture of roof of orbit is:
    A. Blow on back of head
    B. Blow on the forehead
    C. Blow on the parietal bone
    D. Blow on upper jaw.

19. A characterestic finding in direct nasa-orbital-ethmoid fracture is
    A. Telecanthus
    B. Hypoglobus
    C. Infraorbital hypesthesia
    D. Epistaxis.

20. All of the following findings are consistent with an isolated inferior orbital wall fracture and soft issue entrapment except
    A. Subcutaneous emphysema
    B. Infraorbital hypesthesia
    C. Horizontal limitation in ocular motility
    D. Hypoglobus.

21. Orbital roof fractures are characterized by:
    A. Fractures of the orbital floor or medial wall usually occur as well
    B. Tend to occur in adults
    C. The patient must fall from a height greater than 3 m
    D. An upper eyelid hematoma is a common association.

22. A patient sustains blunt trauma to the face. Examination shows enophthalmos, periorbital ecchymosis, subcutaneous emphysema, and ipsilateral epistaxis. These findings are most consistent with a fracture of the:
    A. Anterior wall of the maxillary sinus
    B. Medial wall of the orbit
    C. Nasal bones
    D. Zygomatic arch.

23. A patient is undergoing repair of a comminuted displaced fracture of the left zygoma. Which of the following landmarks will be most useful in restoring the zygoma to its anatomically correct position?
    A. Frontozygomatic suture
    B. Lateral orbital wall
    C. Lateral buttress
    D. Medial buttress.

24. A patient sustains fractures of the right orbit and zygoma in a motor vehicle accident. Which of the following is an indication for immediate ophthalmologic consultation?
    A. Diplopia
    B. Eyelid ptosis
    C. Hyphema
    D. Subconjunctival hemorrhage.

25. A patient is brought to the emergency department following an automobile accident. Examination shows a periorbital hematoma, ophthalmoplegia, ptosis of the upper eyelid, and a fixed dilated pupil on the left. Consensual light reflex is intact. Which of the following is the most likely diagnosis?
    A. Orbital apex syndrome
    B. Retrobulbar hematoma
    C. Superior orbital fissure syndrome
    D. Traumatic mydriasis.

26. A patient sustains a Le Fort I fracture on the left and a Le Fort III fracture on the right in a motor vehicle collision. In this patient, which of the following bones is most likely to be fractured on both sides of the face?
    A. Ethmoid
    B. Palate
    C. Pterygoid plate
    D. Zygoma.

27. A young boy presents with a history of fall from a bicycle. A CT scan showed a pure blowout fracture of the left orbital floor with a slight dislocation of the orbital contents. The indication to repair this orbital blowout fracture includes which one of the following:
    A. Fracture involving less than half of the orbital floor
    B. No inferior rectus entrapment
    C. Inferior rectus weakness
    D. Pain and oculocardiac reflex on upgaze.

28. Surgical incisions to repair orbital floor fractures include all except:
    A. Lower eyelid crease incision
    B. Lower fornix incision
    C. Subciliary incision
    D. Grey line incision.

29. Implants used for orbital fracture repair include all except:
    A. Supramid
    B. Porous polyethylene
    C. Titanium
    D. PMMA.

30. Implants used for orbital fracture repair include all except:
    A. Silicone
    B. PTFE

C. Bone graft

D. Gelfoam.

31. Complete release of entrapped muscle is confirmed by all except:
    A. Hess screen
    B. Diplopia chart
    C. Forced duction test
    D. Electromyography.

32. By definition, all Le Fort fractures must extend posteriorly through the
    A. Pterygoid plates
    B. Maxillary bone
    C. Zygomaticomaxillary complex
    D. Naso-orbital-ethmoidal.

33. The optimal time for surgical repair of orbital floor fractures is generally considered to be
    A. Within 24 hours of injury
    B. 1–3 days following injury
    C. 7–14 days following injury
    D. 2–6 weeks following injury.

34. Regarding surgical repair of a cut canaliculus:
    A. After surgical repair, stents are left in place for 3 weeks
    B. Direct suturing of the cut ends is required
    C. Irrigation using methylene blue may facilitate intraoperative visualization
    D. Repair of all such injuries is recommended.

35. In Traumatic telecanthus, reattachment of the medial canthal tendon to which of the following structures is necessary for reconstruction of the normal eyelid anatomy?
    A. Medial orbital tubercle
    B. Anterior process of the maxilla
    C. Anterior lacrimal crest
    D. Posterior lacrimal crest.

36. The most common cause of indirect traumatic optic neuropathy is blunt trauma to which bone?
    A. Maxillary
    B. Zygomatic
    C. Frontal
    D. Temporal.

37. Which of the following is least likely to be associated with a zygomaticomaxillary complex fracture?

A. Inferior rectus entrapment

B. Trismus

C. Globe ptosis

D. Lateral canthal dystopia.

38. Which of the following findings is most commonly associated with orbital floor fractures?
    A. Orbital cellulitis
    B. Enophthalmos within 24 hours of the fracture
    C. Rapid improvement in traumatic diplopia over a 24-hour period
    D. Unilateral midfacial sensory loss (V2 distribution unilaterally).

39. A patient is seen 2 months after blunt trauma to the right orbit. The examination is normal except for blepharoptosis on the right side. Levator function is normal on both sides, and the patient states the eyelid positions were equal on both sides prior to the injury. There is no enophthalmos or diplopia. What is the best next step in managing this patient?
    A. Surgical exploration and repair of the levator aponeurosis
    B. Close observation with no plan for surgical correction until 3 to 6 months after initial injury
    C. Computed tomography (CT) scan to rule out an orbital fracture
    D. A Tensilon test to rule out new-onset myasthenia gravis.

40. You are asked to see a patient with noninfected second-degree burns to the eyelids. The emergency room physicians ask what topical medicine should be placed over the burns to prevent scarring. What would the most appropriate response be?
    A. Gentamicin in a water-miscible base
    B. Silver sulfadiazine 1% cream
    C. No topical medications
    D. Hydrocortisone 1% ointment.

41. A patient is evaluated for trauma to the right orbit. He has marked proptosis and an intraocular pressure of 40 mm Hg on the affected side. A CT scan shows intraorbital hemorrhage. Which of the following actions would be the least effective in acutely reducing intraocular pressure?

A. Lateral canthotomy and cantholysis

B. Administration of high-dose oral corticosteroids

C. Administration of topical aqueous suppressants

D. Administration of intravenous mannitol.

42. A young boy sustained a right upper eyelid laceration after falling from his bicycle. The laceration measures 15 mm and extends from the eyelid margin to above the eyelid crease. There is an avulsed avascular section of the laceration superiorly. The results of his ocular examination are normal except for marked swelling of the eyelid. What would the least appropriate action in the management of this case be?

A. Check the tetanus status

B. Discard the avulsed tissue

C. Repair the eyelid margin

D. Check the status of the levator muscle.

43. What is the best way to distinguish a restrictive motility disorder from a paretic disorder after a blowout fracture?

A. Alternate prism cover testing

B. Goldmann single binocular visual fields

C. Motility examination of the cardinal positions of gaze

D. Forced-duction testing.

44. Which of the following is not a common sign of an orbital blowout fracture?

A. Tenderness over the zygomaticofrontal suture

B. Infraorbital hypoesthesia

C. Restriction of supraduction

D. Enophthalmos.

45. What type of orbital blow-out fracture requires urgent referral?

A. Medial wall fractures

B. Fractures involving more than 4 mm of displacement

C. Small symptomatic fractures in patients younger than age 18 years

D. Fractures associated with a blood-filled maxillary sinus.

46. Which of the following is the most common indication for repair of medial orbital wall fractures?

A. Epiphora

B. Entrapped muscle

C. Sinusitis

D. Enophthalmos.

47. If a patient has a ruptured globe in addition to a symptomatic blowout fracture, what should the surgeon do?

A. Repair both injuries at the same time

B. Repair the ruptured globe immediately and delay the floor exploration for 2 to 4 weeks

C. Repair the ruptured globe immediately and delay the floor exploration for 2 days

D. Wait 48 hours and then repair both injuries at the same time.

48. A patient has sustained blunt facial and orbital trauma in a motor vehicle accident. The patient has limited supraduction and marked upper eyelid edema and ptosis. A CT scan shows a frontal sinus fracture, orbital roof fracture, and pneumocephalus. What would the appropriate course of action be?

A. Neurosurgical consultation to rule out intracranial injury

B. Valsalva to evaluate brain-orbit interface

C. Forced-duction testing to rule out superior rectus muscle entrapment

D. Superior orbitotomy to rule out a levator laceration.

49. Arteriovenous fistulas that affect the orbit most commonly develop following what type of trauma?

A. Orbital blowout fracture

B. Frontal sinus fracture

C. Penetrating intacranial trauma

D. Basal skull fracture.

50. Limited downgaze is noted in a patient with a known floor fracture. What is the most likely cause of the downgaze deficit?

A. Disinsertion of the inferior rectus muscle from the globe

B. Orbital edema or hemorrhage affecting the inferior rectus muscle

C. Entrapment of the inferior oblique muscle in the floor fracture

D. Concomitant orbital roof fracture with entrapment of the superior rectus muscle.

51. Regarding orbital floor fractures, which is incorrect:
    A. Associated with enophthalmos demand immediate repair
    B. Of the medial wall are associated with orbital emphysema
    C. Associated with hypesthesia of the cheek and upper gum suggest infraorbital nerve damage
    D. Associated with a positive forced duction test always have extraocular muscle entrapped in the fracture.

52. Naso-orbital-ethmoidal fracture is commonly associated with:
    A. Epiphora
    B. Infraorbital nerve hyposthesia
    C. Facial nerve paralysis
    D. Trismus.

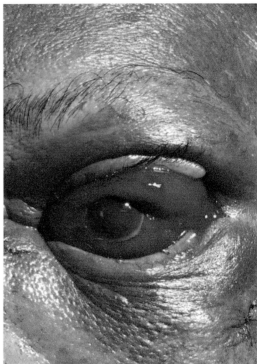

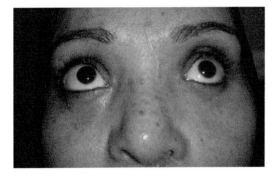

53. Management of the above picture may require all except:
    A. Transnasal wiring
    B. Y miniplate
    C. DCR
    D. Lacrimal stenting.

54. Indications for performing the above procedure include all except:
    A. Hyphema
    B. RAPD
    C. Pulsating retinal vessels
    D. Elevated IOP.

55. The most important step in repair of a cut canaliculus is:
    A. Suturing both ends together
    B. Insertion of a stent
    C. Identification of the distal segment
    D. Using general anesthesia.

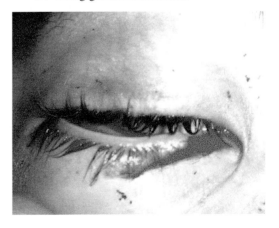

56. The above injury may require the use of all except:
    A. Dye
    B. Local anesthesia
    C. Stent
    D. Vesicoelastic.

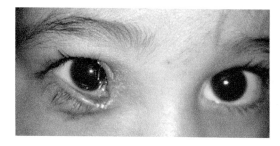

57. Repair of the above post traumatic lesion may require all except:
    A. Wiring
    B. Bony fixation
    C. Lacrimal stent
    D. Using a flap.

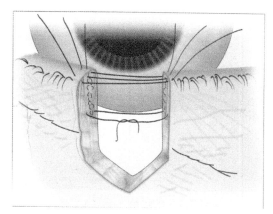

58. The three sutures used in the diagram lies at the level of all except:
    A. Lash line
    B. Grey line
    C. Meibomian orifices
    D. Muco-cutaneous junction.

59. Bad repair of the above injury can result in all except:
    A. Lagophthalmos
    B. Ectropion
    C. Conjunctival shortening
    D. Lid notching.

60. In adults: the preferred anesthesia used in repair of lid injuries is:
    A. Topical
    B. Local
    C. Regional
    D. General.

61. Regarding eyebrow injuries:
    A. Are repaired after lid injuries
    B. Are repaired before forehead injuries
    C. Usually heal well without scarring
    D. Always require tattooing later.

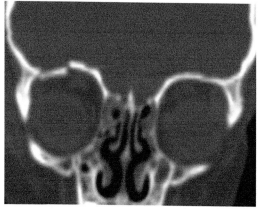

62. Management of this injury is;
    A. Observation
    B. Immediate repair
    C. Repair within 48 hours
    D. Repair within 2 weeks.

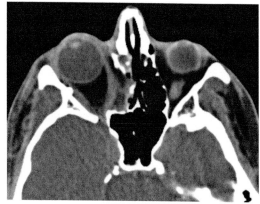

63. Features of this lesion includes all except:
    A. Subcutaneous emphysema
    B. Epistaxis

C. Hypesthesia

D. Diplopia.

64. Indications to remove an orbital FB include all except:

A. Organic nature

B. Close to the optic nerve

C. Associated with diplopia

D. Anterior.

65. In acute severe traumatic optic neuropathy (TON) associated with major head trauma, which of the following statements is most likely to be true?

A. Computed tomography (CT) of the optic canal is commonly abnormal

B. Fundoscopy is commonly abnormal

C. High-dose steroids are indicated

D. Intervention is unlikely to result in improvement.

66. Which individual variable at presentation is the strongest predictor of visual outcome using the ocular trauma score (OTS)?

A. Endophthalmitis

B. Globe rupture

C. Presence of relative afferent pupillary defect

D. Visual acuity.

Answers of Trauma

1	B	21	D	41	B	61	B
2	D	22	B	42	B	62	A
3	C	23	B	43	D	63	C
4	B	24	C	44	A	64	B
5	D	25	C	45	C	65	D
6	D	26	C	46	B	66	D
7	B	27	D	47	B		
8	D	28	D	48	A		
9	C	29	D	49	D		
10	B	30	D	50	B		
11	A	31	D	51	D		
12	B	32	A	52	A		
13	D	33	C	53	D		
14	C	34	D	54	A		
15	A	35	D	55	C		
16	B	36	C	56	B		
17	C	37	A	57	D		
18	B	38	D	58	D		
19	A	39	B	59	C		
20	C	40	C	60	C		

The Orbit

8

Essam A. El Toukhy

The orbit is defined by the four bony walls surrounding the eye and all of the contents contained within that space. Understanding the anatomy of the relevant nerves, extraocular muscles, vascular system, adipose tissue, lacrimal system, lymphatics, and anterior segment structures in addition to the adjacent nasal sinuses and cranial cavity is a must. Orbital pathology can be caused by any process that involves these structures, as well as distant disease processes including metastasis or causing inflammation of the orbit. The examination will allow the oculoplastic surgeon to form a differential diagnosis that will often be refined by imaging and laboratory studies. Categories include vascular, inflammatory, traumatic, autoimmune, metabolic, infectious, neoplastic, congenital, and endocrine.

For many general ophthalmologists, the orbital evaluation may seem to involve structures that are away from a general ophthalmologist's usual structures. However, an organized approach to the exam will make this area feel familiar.

Proptosis is the commonest orbital manifestation. The ophthalmologist should always check vision, pupils, pressures, confrontation visual fields, and eye movements.

Pain is another common manifestation. The *level, character, onset and progression* of the pain are helpful in determining the etiology of the orbital process. Pain is most commonly caused by inflammation, either autoimmune or infectious. Orbital inflammatory disease and orbital cellulitis are examples of these processes. Both processes cause pain via the inflammatory cascade. This is why orbital inflammatory syndrome is sometimes difficult to differentiate from orbital cellulitis when both are unilateral and causing pain. Cellulitis will be associated with malaise, and a leukocytosis in most cases. Benign processes generally do not cause pain. Large slow growing benign masses typically do not cause severe pain, but a large mass may cause a pressure type or discomfort. Chronic orbital processes include thyroid eye disease (by far the most common cause of proptosis), sarcoidosis and granulomatosis with polyangiitis. Thyroid eye disease typically has an indefinite onset and is slowly progressive over weeks and months. Malignant tumors, late in the course, can invade sensory nerves and cause pain associated with hypesthesia. In some cases the proptosis may be present for years, progress very slowly, and cause no pain (benign mixed tumor of the lacrimal gland).

Past medical history can be helpful. A history of any cancer should alert the physician to the possibility of a metastasis with lung, breast, colon, and prostate cancer being the

E. A. El Toukhy (✉)
Oculoplasty Service, Cairo University, Cairo, Egypt
e-mail: eeltoukhy@yahoo.com

© The Author(s), under exclusive license to Springer Nature Switzerland AG 2021
E. A. El Toukhy (ed.), *Oculoplasty for Ophthalmologists*, https://doi.org/10.1007/978-3-030-68469-3_8

most common. Previous surgery and trauma also notably affect the orbital structures allowing physicians to contextualize any proptosis measured.

An appropriate physical exam includes slit lamp evaluation of the anterior segment and all the usual components of a complete eye exam. Unique to the orbital exam is the evaluation of proptosis, periorbital changes, palpation, and detection of globe pulsation.

Gross proptosis or prominent eyes will be immediately obvious and probably indicates that the individual has asymmetry outside of the range of normal. Quantification of this finding is performed using the Hertel exophthalmometer. A normal range is about 18 mm.

The most important component of measurement is asymmetry between the two eyes. A measurement of the tip of the cornea to the lateral orbital rim differing more than 2 mm between the two eyes should be considered abnormal. Even in the absence of pain, progression, or relevant past medical history, incidental asymmetry of the orbits that is greater than 2 mm should be investigated further with imaging if progression is observed. Asymmetry and progression are the greatest red flags for proptosis.

The types of globe displacement also add additional clues to the etiology of an orbital process. A slow-growing tumor within the muscle cone will cause axial proptosis, meaning the eye will be pushed directly forward out of the socket. Masses within the extraconal spaces result in displacement of the globe away from a mass. A superior mass will result in inferior displacement of the globe. Lacrimal gland tumors result in inferior and possibly medial displacement of the globe. An exception to this rule is the scirrhous carcinoma breast cancer metastasis. The sclerosing tumor can cause enophthalmos. Lateral displacement of the globe is typically seen in sinus disease including carcinoma or a mucocele. Superior displacement of the globe is relatively rare, but may occur from maxillary sinus tumor. Interestingly, the most common inferior orbital mass is lymphoma, despite the fact that most lymphomas arise in the superior orbit.

Most periorbital changes can be identified using a pen light. The pen light can help illuminate suspicious skin lesions, check the pupils, and assess the eye movements including the eyelid excursion. This quick exam would allow to identify retraction of the upper eyelids showing exposed sclera above the limbus, lid lagophthalmos in downgaze and temporal flare, all caused by thyroid eye disease. Other pathognomonic findings include fullness of the temple in sphenoid wing meningioma, an S-shaped eyelid in a patient with neurofibromatosis type 1 with a plexiform neurofibroma, or a diabetic patient with routine orbital cellulitis that have a necrotic black lesion in the nasopharynx indicating a phycomycosis. During slit lamp examination we may identify a salmon colored patch of the conjunctiva confirming diagnosis of lymphoma of the orbit. During fundus examination we may see ciliary shunt vessels of the optic nerve, consistent with an orbital meningioma, or the "candle wax dripping" periphlebitis associated with sarcoidosis.

Palpation of the orbit may identify a specific mass or a general fullness of the orbit (resistance to retropulsion). Note the position and character of any masses. A child presenting with a slow growing superotemporal, discrete, smooth mass likely has a dermoid cyst. Upon palpation of the skin overlying the lacrimal gland, the patient may note some diminished sensation. This hypesthesia is associated with lacrimal gland malignancies deriving from the lacrimal gland epithelium. The ophthalmologist may identify the heat and pain due to orbital inflammation or infection, associated with the redness that was noted on inspection. Any possible restriction of extraocular muscles identified on exam can be further tested with forced ductions.

Pulsation is a sign suggesting a pulsatile vascular lesion such as an AVM or high flow carotid cavernous fistula. It may also be seen after the removal of the orbital roof or lateral wall following a sphenoid wing meningioma excision. Auscultation can also be applied to the globe and orbit where a high-flow fistula may produce a bruit, typically accompanied by dilated episcleral vessels.

The Various Orbital Diagnoses Include

Vascular

Many vascular pathologies affect the orbit. In children, the infantile hemangioma usually appears in the first few weeks of life. These hemangiomas grow over a period of several weeks and involute to a degree over 5–10 years. In contrast to this childhood vascular lesion, adults may present with slowly progressive axial proptosis due to a cavernous vascular malformation in the muscle cone. Following trauma, a direct high flow carotid cavernous fistula can occur, typically of acute or subacute onset associated with pain. Accompanying symptoms usually include high intraocular pressure, unilateral proptosis, and acute progression. Indirect fistulas can occur spontaneously in older adults. These have low flow and are more likely to have normal intraocular pressure and slower progression without a bruit.

Infection

Orbital bacterial cellulitis presents acutely with pain, unilateral proptosis, and rapid progression. There is tenderness on palpation with notable edema and erythema, often with induration. Fungal cellulitis occurs in immunosuppressed patients. The inadequate immune response allows the normally docile fungus to infect the orbital tissues. In this case, typical signs of orbital inflammation are not present due to the lack of normal immunocompetency.

Trauma

Proptosis resulting from trauma is caused by a retrobulbar hematoma resulting in pain of rapid onset with periorbital ecchymosis, edema, chemosis, and vision loss due to high intraocular pressure or stretching of the optic nerve if severe.

Autoimmune

This etiology includes the continuum of idiopathic orbital inflammatory syndrome to IgG antibody-mediated inflammatory disease. It occurs and typically results in unilateral proptosis with pain, acute onset, chemosis and injection, a lack of response to antibiotics, and rapid improvement with high-dose oral steroids. In contrast to this immune related process, thyroid eye disease presents less acutely, over weeks with slowly progressive signs of inflammation, eyelid retraction and possible motility disturbance and proptosis.

Metabolic

In rare instances, fluid shifts in burn victims can result in orbital compartment syndrome following aggressive IV rehydration, resulting in a similar picture as that of a retrobulbar hematoma.

Iatrogenic

Surprisingly some proptosis can be purposeful and beneficial cosmetically. Orbital volume augmentation with implants or fillers can restore ocular prominence. Intraorbital implants are commonly used to restore symmetry. Filler is rarely used to improve enophthalmos.

Neoplasm

Benign and metastatic tumors vary significantly in their presentation. Pleomorphic adenoma of the lacrimal gland may slowly progress over many months to result in non-axial inferonasal displacement of the globe while rhabdomyosarcoma in a child could have an aggressive orbital cellulitis-type presentation with onset over days. Differentiation within the category of neoplasm typically requires imaging.

Congenital

A dermoid cyst can be differentiated from an encephalocele by location and progression. Most dermoid cysts arise laterally from within the frontozygomatic suture. Encephaloceles are present medially and often increase with the Valsalva maneuver.

Endocrine

Thyroid eye disease (TED) is an autoimmune and endocrine related disease due to its antibody acting directly on fibroblasts that result in fibrosis of muscles and differentiation into adipocytes in the orbit. It is the most common cause of bilateral and unilateral proptosis in adults, which typically presents bilaterally with many periorbital changes including eyelid retraction, eyelid flare, proptosis, and has both an acute and chronic form.

Imaging of the orbit is often indicated for further evaluation of proptosis. Radiological imaging is an essential diagnostic tool in the oculoplastic specialty, particularly in orbital and lacrimal lesions as the pathology cannot be visualized from outside. Moreover, it can be used in the management plan and follow up of the patients.

Imaging Modalities

1. Ultrasound (US)
Ultrasound (US) with Doppler can be used in the diagnosis and follow up of various globe and orbital lesions. It is the first imaging modality in children with superficial lesions. The technique is non-invasive, cost-effective and easy to perform, and has a high accuracy for the characterization of vascular lesions. However, it is operator dependent and cannot visualize the orbit completely. Also, it is contraindicated if rupture globe is suspected.

2. Computed Tomography
CT is the initial imaging modality for the evaluation of orbital trauma; infection and detection of a foreign body. It is superior to MRI in the detection of calcification, or acute hemorrhage; evaluation of orbital osseous lesions; as well as the assessment of orbital soft-tissue lesion with suspicion of bony erosion. CT is preferred in the setting of an emergency or if there is a contraindication for MR examination.

Thin slice multi-detector CT scan of the orbit provides rapid volumetric image acquisitions. Coronal and sagittal reconstructed images are routinely obtained in bone and soft tissue windows. 3D reconstructed images are beneficial in the assessment of complex orbital fractures, orbito-cranial masses, fibrous dysplasia or neurofibromatosis.

CT scan of the orbits is usually performed following the intravenous (IV) administration of an iodinated contrast medium in the venous phase. Contrast-enhanced CT examination is indicated if an orbital mass is suspected to allow differentiation of different orbital lesions according to their enhancement pattern. Non-contrast CT examination is performed in cases for orbital trauma or thyroid orbitopathy as these pathologies are very well delineated by hypodense orbital fat.

It is crucial to note that, CT of the orbits is not performed both without and with contrast administration; as it does not yield significant diagnostic improvement, with the risk of doubling the radiation dose to the lens.

The eye is a sensitive organ to radiation, and exposure to higher doses of radiation may lead to the development of early cataract. The risk of radiation exposure is especially important in the pediatric patients with special attention in children having malignant lesions who require long-term follow-up imaging to assess response after therapy and to diagnose early recurrence.

CT angiography (CTA) and CT venography (CTV) are helpful for assessment of orbital vascular lesions. Also, it can be useful in planning further evaluation and management of these lesions.

3. Magnetic Resonance Imaging
MRI is the modality of choice for evaluating most of the orbital lesions, particularly in non-emergency settings, with imaging of patients presenting with subacute or chronic symptoms.

MRI has higher soft tissue resolution and tissue characterization compared to CT and provides more precise delineation of the different orbital compartments. Thus, MRI is preferred in the evaluation of suspected orbit neoplasms, orbit inflammatory disorders, orbit vascular malformations, and optic nerve sheath complex lesions. Moreover, MR is ideal for visualization of intracranial extension of orbital lesions, as well as lesions at the orbital apex, optic canal and cavernous sinus.

However, MR is more expensive with longer examination time compared to CT. It requires sedation in some patients; additionally, it is contraindicated in patients with a cardiac pacemaker, aneurysmal clip, or metallic foreign bodies.

The standard protocol for MRI orbit examination is to acquire both unenhanced and enhanced imaging after IV administration of gadolinium contrast medium. Unenhanced MRI examination is performed alone, if there is a contraindication to gadolinium IV administration like renal failure, contrast allergy or pregnancy.

MRA and MRV examinations can be used in imaging of orbital vascular lesions; however, they are more susceptible to artifacts and lower spatial resolution than CTA and CTV studies. However, they can be done without contrast medium, with no risk of ionizing radiation, thus they can be used in patients who cannot tolerate iodinated contrast material.

Diffusion-weighted imaging (DWI) is based upon assessing the random Brownian motion of water molecules within the tissue. A lesion with high cellularity demonstrates restricted diffusion and low apparent diffusion coefficient (ADC) value. The use of DWI has been reported to further increase the diagnostic utility of MRI in the characterization of orbital masses. Tumors composed of tightly packed cells with a high nuclear-to-cytoplasmic ratio like lymphoma show restricted diffusion. Additionally, DWI is valuable in differentiating abscess from other inflammatory processes as the thick purulent material in an abscess demonstrates diffusion restriction.

4. Conventional Angiography

Conventional *angiography* has advantages over CTA and MRA examinations, as it is real-time imaging that provides better temporal resolution with evaluation of blood flow dynamics.

However, because of its invasive nature, it is only indicated in selected cases. It is used as a problem- solving tool when the findings of initial CT or MR angiography examination are unclear. Also, it provides intra-procedural guidance of endovascular treatment.

Before we review any type of scan, consider your original exam. When the patient has globe displacement, investigate the area of the scan where we could imagine a mass pushing the globe. If we have identified a mass, then the next consideration is if it is discrete or infiltrative. Erosion of the bone is more indicative of a malignant process. A fossa that is formed from a mass or from the pressure of long-standing thyroid eye disease is indicative of a chronic process and usually represents a benign process. Generally smaller lesions are better lesions but are not necessarily prognostic. Therefore, a small, well circumscribed, homogeneous, mass indenting but not eroding the bone is likely a benign process. Most other tumors and masses are diagnosed with incisional biopsy except where removal of the entire lesion is easier such as a cavernous hemangioma or a dermoid cyst. A "biopsy" in those cases would be curative for both lesions. The incisional biopsy allows for minimal damage to surrounding structures while providing specific information or further non-surgical intervention including radiation, chemotherapy, and the more recent treatment of checkpoint inhibitors. A growing list of targets allows the native host immune system to attack cancer cells with a high degree of specificity based on tissue DNA testing. This has resulted in multiple cases that in previous decades would have been treated only with exenteration but can now be approached differently.

The Orbit

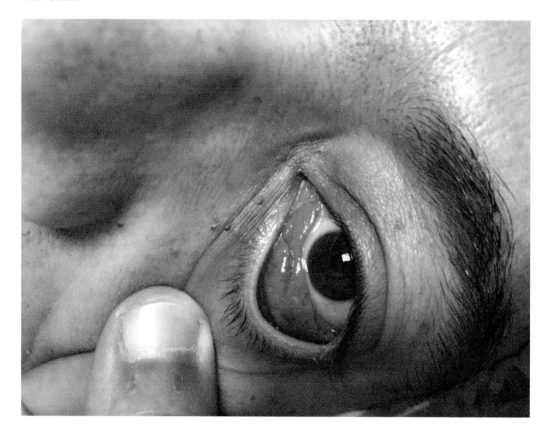

1. This lesion is characteristic for:
   A. Leukemia
   B. Lymphoma
   C. Sarcoidosis
   D. Steven Johnson syndrome.

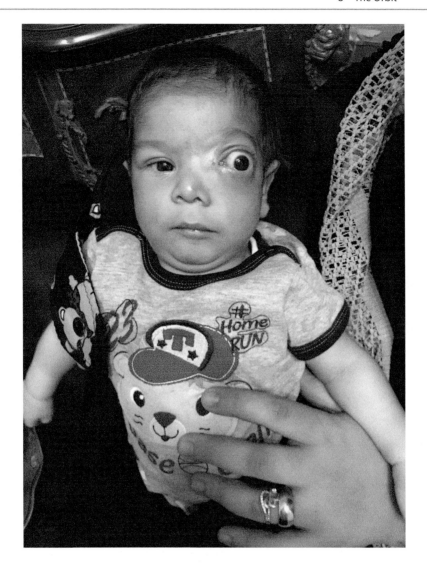

2. The child has proptosis directed down and
   out. Possibilities include all except:
   A. Mucocele
   B. Meningocele
   C. Dacryocele
   D. Subperiosteal abscess.

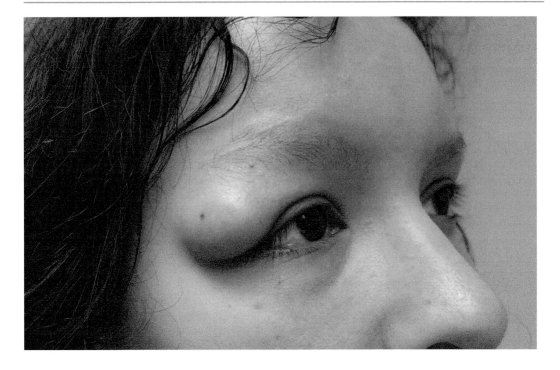

3. The above lesion is:
    A. Rhabdomyosarcoma
    B. Dermoid cyst

C. Hemangioma
D. Mucocele.

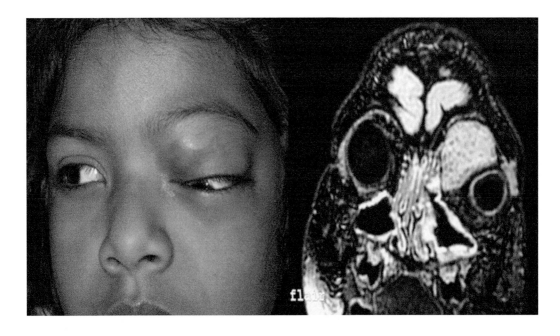

4. The above lesion is:
    A. Rhabdomyosarcoma
    B. Dermoid cyst

C. Hemangioma
D. Mucocele.

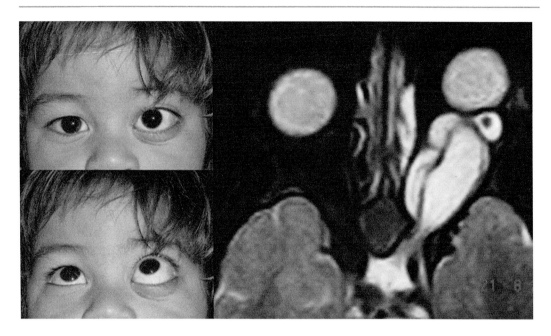

5. The above lesion is:
   A. Rhabdomyosarcoma
   B. Optic nerve glioma
   C. Cavernous hemangioma
   D. Optic nerve meningioma.

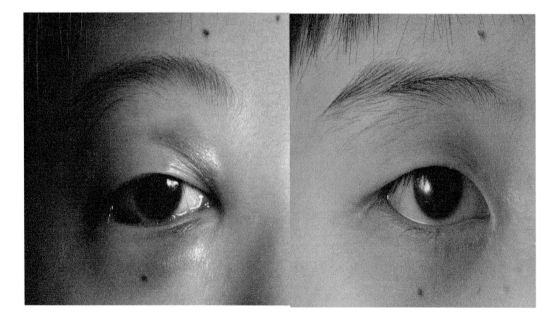

6. The above lesion enlarges during upper respiratory tract infections. The most probable diagnosis is:
   A. Hemangioma
   B. Lymphangioma
   C. Hemangiopericytoma
   D. Lymphoma.

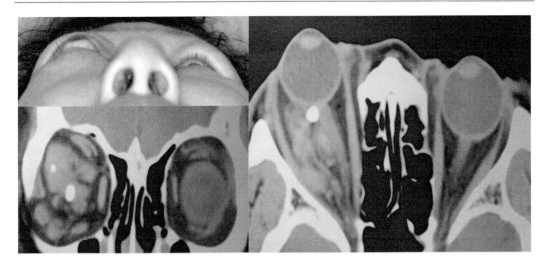

7. The hyperdense lesion in the CT points to
   the diagnosis of:
   A. Hemangioma

B. Lymphangioma
C. Hemangiopericytoma
D. Venous malformation.

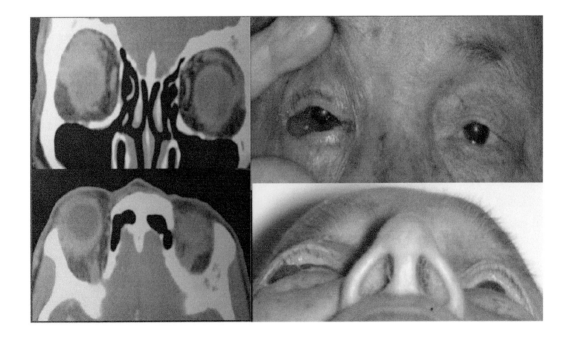

8. The above lesion is characteristic of:
   A. Thyroid ophthalmopathy
   B. Idiopathic orbital inflammation

C. Orbital cellulitis
D. Cavernous sinus thrombosis.

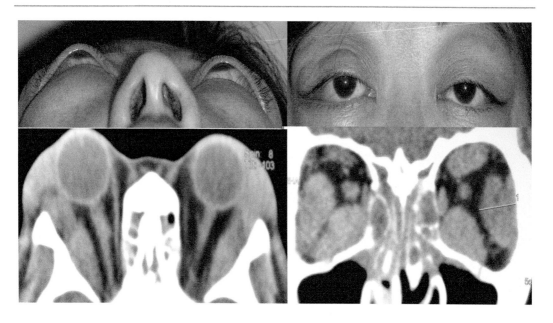

9. The above lesion is characteristic of:
   A. Thyroid ophthalmopathy
   B. Idiopathic orbital inflammation

C. IgG4 orbital inflammation
D. Cavernous sinus thrombosis.

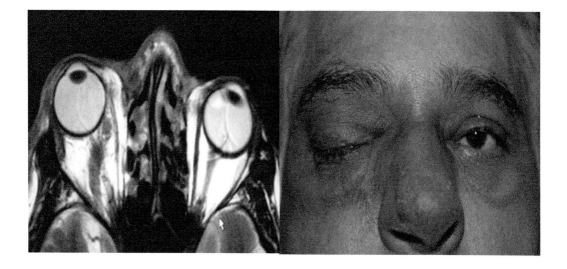

10. The enlarged superior ophthalmic vein points to the diagnosis of:
    A. Thyroid ophthalmopathy

B. Idiopathic orbital inflammation
C. IgG4 orbital inflammation
D. Cavernous sinus thrombosis.

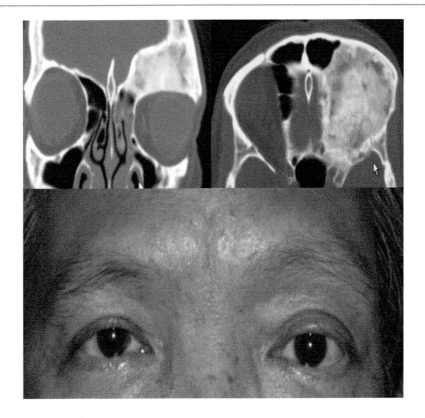

11. The above lesion is characteristic of:
    A. Frontal sinus mucocele
    B. Lacrimal gland tumor
    C. Fibrous dysplasia
    D. Eosinophlic granuloma.

12. Regarding micophthalmia, one is false
    A. All children with micophthalmia have hypoplastic orbit
    B. Most microphthalmic eyes have no potential for vision
    C. Enucleation is nessesary for fitting of ocular prosthesis
    D. Dermis fat graft may grow resulting in progressive socket expansion.

13. A patient with subperiosteal abscess can be managed by observation in the following situation except:
    A. Patient younger than 9 years
    B. Medial location of subperiosteal abscess
    C. Presence of gas in the abscess on CT scan
    D. Associated with isolated ethimoidal sinusitis.

14. Orbital tuberculosis, one is false:
    A. Usually unilateral
    B. Mimic orbital malignancy
    C. Chronic drainage fistula may be the presenting sign
    D. Treated surgically.

15. Regarding orbital decompression in thyroid eye disease, one is false:
    A. Indicated to restore globe position even if there is no sight threatening conditions
    B. Indicated if radiotherapy was not effective
    C. Fat versus bone decompression is based on patient's age
    D. Orbital surgery should precede strabismus surgery.

16. During decompression of orbital floor, diplopia and dystopia can be minimized by preserving:
    A. The palatine bone
    B. The bone between the medial wall and the floor
    C. The zygomatic bone
    D. The ethmoidal bone.

17. Nonspecific orbital inflammation, one is false:
    A. The muscle insertion is involved in 50% of cases
    B. The ring sign in B-scan ultrasound indicates presence of posterior scleritis
    C. Rapid and favorable response to steroid indicates a cell mediated pathology
    D. It is a diagnosis of exclusion.

18. Clinical features of nonspecific orbital inflammation in children, one is false:
    A. One third of cases are bilateral
    B. Mostly associated with systemic disorders
    C. Headache and abdominal pain are a common finding
    D. Uveitis maybe the presenting sign.

19. Clinical features of infantile capillary hemangioma, one is false:
    A. Start to involute after the first year of life
    B. More common in females
    C. MRI finding show intralesional vascular channels with low blood flow
    D. Can be a part of Kasabach–Merritt syndrome.

20. The management paradigram for infantile capillary hemangioma include, one is false:
    A. Beta blockers
    B. Systemic steroids
    C. Sclerosing agents
    D. Surgery.

21. Regarding cavernous hemangioma, one is false:
    A. The most common benign neoplasm of the orbit in adult females
    B. May present with increased intraocular pressure
    C. Arteriography and venography are not useful in the diagnosis
    D. Radiodense phlebliths are present in early growing lesions.

22. Features of hemangiopericytoma, one is false:
    A. It is a hypercellular and hypervascular mass lesions
    B. Benign lesions may recur and metastasize

    C. There is a strong correlation between mitotic rates and the clinical behaviors
    D. It appears as a bluish encapsulated mass during surgery.

23. True statement regarding lymphatic malformation(lymphangioma) is:
    A. Present since birth
    B. Contain both arterial and lymphatic component
    C. Does not proliferate
    D. Intralesional sclerosing agents have no role in management.

24. The best treatment for a patient with decreased visual acuity due to optic sheath meningioma that does not extend outside the orbit is:
    A. Systemic corticosteroid
    B. Fractional stereotactic radiation
    C. Proton pump radiation
    D. Exenteration.

25. The best approach to an intraconal orbital tumor is:
    A. Trans caruncular orbitotomy
    B. Vertical eye lid splitting orbitotomy
    C. Medial orbitotomy
    D. Lateral orbitotomy.

26. Regarding exenteration, one is false:
    A. Considered in management of recurrent non responding rhabdomyosarcoma to radio and chemotherapy
    B. Total exenteration is the removal of all intraorbital soft tissue with or without the skin of eye lids
    C. Fixating of ossoointegrated implant is achieved with glue
    D. The exenteration prosthesis usually do not blink or move.

27. Regarding exophthalmometer the most appropriate statement is:
    A. Is not useful in pulsatile proptosis
    B. Normal distance between the apex of the cornea and lateral orbital wall rim is <20 mm
    C. A difference between the two eyes of <4 mm is considered normal
    D. Most common cause of bilateral proptosis is orbital pseudotumor.

28. Regarding the anatomy of the optic canal one of the following statement is true:
    A. Entrance to the optic canal lies inside annulus of Zinn.
    B. Medial wall of the canal is the medial wall of the sphenoid.
    C. Optic nerve leave the optic canal to enter the anterior cranial fossa
    D. Optic nerve injury is due to absence of periorbita in the canal.

29. Good reflectivity and dancing spikes along with good sound transmission is seen in orbital B-scan in which tumor?
    A. Cavernous haemangioma
    B. Pleomorphic adenoma
    C. Adenoid cystic carcinoma
    D. Lipodermoid.

30. What is the volume of the orbit?
    A. 10 ml
    B. 20 ml
    C. 30 ml
    D. 50 ml.

31. One of the following statements is incorrect regarding the orbital septum:
    A. Is separated from the levator aponeurosis by orbital fat
    B. Is firmly attached to Whitnall's ligament
    C. Fuses with the capsulopalpebral fascia in the lower lid
    D. Inserts on the levator aponeurosis about 3–5 mm above the tarsal plate.

32. In the management of malignant lacrimal gland tumor the least appropriate statement is:
    A. Percutaneous biopsy is contraindicated
    B. Perineural extension into the cavernous sinus is common
    C. Surgical debulking with intracarotid chemotherapy is an option
    D. Exenteration is required.

33. One of the following is true regarding osteoma:
    A. Premalignant tumor
    B. Originates from mesodermal tissue
    C. Rapidly growing tumor
    D. Surgical excision is the first line of management.

34. Mucosa associated lymphoid tissue (MALT):
    A. Accounts for less than 10% of orbital lymphoma
    B. Possible association with chronic chlamydia infection
    C. Has no malignant potential
    D. Systemic association is rare.

35. Regarding the orbital wall structure the most appropriate statement is:
    A. The orbital roof is made of the frontal bone and ethmoidal bone
    B. Separates the anterior cranial fossa from the orbit
    C. The superior orbital fissure is bounded superiorly by the lesser wing of the sphenoid
    D. The optic canal transmits the ophthalmic vein.

36. Regarding orbital metastatic tumors in adults, the least likely statement is:
    A. Breast and lung cancer account for the majority of orbital metastases
    B. Pain is a frequent presentation
    C. 75% of patients have a history of known primary tumor
    D. Extraocular muscle involvement is rare.

37. Which is the most common orbital encapsulated tumor?
    A. Lacrimal gland tumor
    B. Cavernous haemangioma
    C. Intraorbital dermoid cyst
    D. Lymphangioma.

38. Management of Rhabdomyosarcoma in a 6 years old boy usually involves which one of the following?
    A. Enucleation and orbital radiation
    B. Lumbar puncture to rule out central nervous system metastasis
    C. Systemic chemotherapy and orbital radiation
    D. Exenteration of the orbit.

39. Which one of the following statements is true in regards to unilateral exophthalmos in a child?
    A. Capillary hemangiomas are the most common benign primary orbital tumors in children

B. Optic nerve meningiomas are more common than gliomas in children
C. Neurofibroma is the malignant tumor that most commonly produces exophthalmos in children
D. Thyroid ophthalmopathy is the most common cause of unilateral exophthalmos in children.

40. Examination of a 70-year-old patient with a progressively enlarging mass in the left inferior orbit reveals a "salmon patch" appearance of the inferior fornix. The most likely diagnosis is:
    A. Melanoma
    B. Sebaceous carcinoma
    C. Lymphoma
    D. Reactive lymphoid hyperplasia.

41. A 1-year-old girl with a round, well-demarcated mass at the superotemporal rim that has been there since birth. The most likely diagnosis is:
    A. Rhabdomyosarcoma
    B. Capillary hemangiomas
    C. Neurofibroma
    D. Dermoid cyst.

42. A 63-year-old patient has a 3 years history of steadily progressive bilateral painless proptosis and visual loss. Ct scan showed bilateral orbital infiltrates. Biopsy of the orbital infiltrates was reported as "reactive lymphoid hyperplasia." The most appropriate treatment is which one of the following?
    A. Radiation with a dose of 1500–2000 ncGy
    B. Systemic steroids
    C. Complete surgical excision
    D. Systemic chemotherapy.

43. A 56-year-old man presents with bilateral proptosis, double vision and chemosis. Which one of the following features on CT orbits distinguishes thyroid related orbitopathy from orbital inflammatory syndrome?
    A. Periorbital soft tissue edema of the lids
    B. Enlarged extraocular muscle
    C. Absence of a thickened extraocular muscle tendon
    D. Enlarged lacrimal glands.

44. Presence of sudden enophthalmos without history of a previous injury involving the orbit in adults is suspicious for:
    A. Cavernous hemangioma
    B. Orbital cellulitis
    C. Thyroid-related orbitopathy
    D. Metastatic breast cancer in a woman.

45. A 63-year-old diabetic patient presented with pain in the right eye, redness, and swelling one month earlier. Examination revealed severe right proptosis, eyelid edema, limited movement in all directions and necrotic crust and lesions on the hard palate and nasal passages. The proper treatment of this condition includes all of the following EXCEPT:
    A. Radiation of the orbits
    B. Amphotericin B for 6 weeks
    C. Stabilizing the underlying disease process
    D. Debridement of all devitalized tissue, including Exenteration if necessary.

46. A 56-year-old woman presents with bilateral proptosis, double vision, and chemosis. She has bilateral lid retraction and lid lag. The most common recommended surgical order of therapy is:
    A. Orbital decompression, strabismus surgery, and eyelid retraction surgical repair
    B. Eyelid retraction surgery, orbital decompression, and strabismus surgery
    C. Orbital decompression and eyelid retraction surgery repair
    D. Eyelid retraction surgery, strabismus surgery, and orbital decompression.

47. A 55-year-old patient presents with gradual painless proptosis in the left eye. On examination, visual acuity is normal; the left globe is displaced inferiorly and medially and a firm lobular mass is palpated near the superior lateral orbital rim. CT of the left orbit showed a lacrimal gland mass with no bony erosion. The next step in the management of this patient would be:
    A. Incisional biopsy
    B. Metastatic work-up
    C. A 2-week course of systemic corticosteroids
    D. Excisional biopsy.

48. A 10-year-old patient with painless outward protruding of the right eye combined with loss of vision in this eye for 3 months. Which one of the following radiological features is considered pathognomonic for optic nerve glioma?
    A. Multiple cystic cavities within optic nerve
    B. Kinking of the optic nerve
    C. "Tram-track" enlargement of the optic nerve
    D. Adjacent bony erosion.

49. A 36-year-old patient with a presumed diagnosis of Idiopathic Orbital Inflammatory Syndrome (IOIS) was treated with 60 mg of oral prednisone for 2 weeks with no improvement. What would be the next step in the management of this case?
    A. Orbital irradiation
    B. Induction with intravenous methylprednisolone
    C. Oral cyclophosphamide
    D. Orbital biopsy.

50. A 6-year-old boy presents with redness of his left eye. On examination, the skin of the upper and lower eyelid is red and inflamed, no orbital tenderness, visual acuity is normal in both eyes, he is orthotropic in primary position, and Hertel exophthalmometry reads 16 mm in the right eye and 18 mm in the left eye. Which of the following examination findings that best differentiates between the diagnoses of preseptal and orbital cellulitis?
    A. External examination findings (erythema, warmth)
    B. Ocular motility findings
    C. Exophthalmometry
    D. Fever.

51. Which one of the following is NOT a typical manifestation of Idiopathic Orbital Inflammatory Syndrome?
    A. Peripheral ulcerative keratitis
    B. Dacryoadenitis
    C. Orbital myositis
    D. Optic perineuritis.

52. A 70-year-old female, with no history of trauma, complains of mild redness and irritation of her left eye for 2 months. On examination, visual acuity is normal OU; there is 3 mm of proptosis on the left and arterialized conjunctival and episcleral vessels. IOP is 30 mmHg in OS and 12 mmHg in OD. Arterialization of vessels is most likely caused by disturbance in which of the following structure?
    A. Intracranial ophthalmic artery
    B. Intra-orbital central retinal artery
    C. Meningeal branches of Internal Carotid Artery
    D. Cervical common carotid artery.

53. Which of the following is not a major criterion for the diagnostic of Neurofibromatosis type I?
    A. Optic nerve glioma
    B. Lisch nodules
    C. Posterior subcapsular cataract
    D. Plexiform neurofibromas.

54. Surgical spaces of the orbit include all except one:
    A. The sub-periorbital surgical space, which is the potential space between the bone and the periorbita
    B. The extraconal surgical space, which between the periorbita and the muscle cone
    C. The intraconal surgical space, which lies within the muscle cone
    D. Sub-Conjunctival surgical space, which lies between the conjunctiva and the Tenon.

55. Orbital cellulitis, one is false:
    A. Implies active infection of the orbital soft tissue anterior to the orbital septum
    B. 90% of cases of orbital cellulitis occurs as a secondary extension of acute or chronic bacterial sinusitis
    C. Delay in treatment may result in development of cavernous sinus thrombosis
    D. Decreased vision and pupillary abnormalities suggest involvement of orbital apex.

56. Optic nerve gliomas, one is false:
    A. Occur predominantly in children in the second decade of life
    B. The chief clinical feature is gradual, painless unilateral and axial Proptosis

C. In the majority of cases are self- limited and show minimal growth

D. Diagnosis of these tumors can usually be established by orbital CT scan.

57. Regarding Rhabdomyosarcoma, one is true:
    A. The most common secondary orbital malignancy in childhood
    B. The average age of onset is 3 years
    C. The tumour is usually retrobulabar
    D. A biopsy must be done immediately, usually via an anterior orbitotomy.

58. Lacrimal gland tumour, one is false:
    A. Clinically, the large majority of lacrimal gland tumors will represent idiopathic inflammatory disease
    B. Usually are not responding to anti-inflammatory medication
    C. Majority of them do not require surgical intervention
    D. Majority of cases do not require biopsy.

59. Which one of the following statements about capillary hemangiomas is false?
    A. Systemic interferon may lead to involution
    B. They are more common in girls than in boys
    C. They characteristically blanch with pressure
    D. MRI findings show intralesional vascular channels with low blood flow.

60. The epibulbar lesion most commonly seen in children younger than 15 years is:
    A. Dermoid
    B. Pyogenic granuloma
    C. Nevus
    D. Epithelial inclusion cyst.

61. In childhood orbital cellulitis, the least important thing is:
    A. Orbital imaging
    B. Hospitalization
    C. Isolation of the infectious organism
    D. Pediatric ENT consultation.

62. Which of the following statements about optic nerve glioma is false?
    A. The age range with the highest incidence is 2–6 years
    B. Two common means of presentation include visual loss and proptosis

C. The classic radiographic appearance of the lesion on computed tomography (CT) scanning is a fusiform enlargement of the optic nerve

D. Tumors arising from the optic nerve have a poorer prognosis than those arising from the optic chiasm.

63. Which one of the following statements about ocular adnexal dermoid cysts is false?
    A. They are choristomatous arrests of epithelial tissue
    B. The most common location is the superonasal orbital rim
    C. Generally, they do not enlarge after the first year of life
    D. Radiography of orbital lesions generally demonstrates bony excavation.

64. Regarding MRI in orbital disease, one is false:
    A. No view of bone or calcium
    B. Less soft tissue detail
    C. Multiple planes can be imaged at once
    D. Better for orbitocranial junction or intracranial problem.

65. Capillary hemangioma, one is false:
    A. Are common primary benign tumours of the orbit in children
    B. Manifest primarily in the second year of life
    C. The majority of capillary hemangiomas are superficial
    D. Ophthalmic indications for treatment are anismetropia, strabismus and amblyopia.

66. Clinical feature of infantile capillary hemangioma, one is true:
    A. Start to involute about the 3rd year of life
    B. More common in males
    C. MRI finding show intralesional vascular channels with high blood flow
    D. Sclerosing agents are included in the management paradigram.

67. The first line of treatment of optic nerve glioma is:
    A. Observation
    B. Surgical excision
    C. Radiotherapy
    D. Chemotherapy.

68. In the evaluation of a child with unilateral exophthalmos, which assumption is correct:
    A. Cavernous hemangiomas are the most common benign orbital tumour in children
    B. Thyroid ophthalmopathy is the most common cause of unilateral exophthalmos among children
    C. Optic nerve meningiomas are more common than gliomas in children
    D. Proptosis is an unusual presentation of nonspecific orbital inflammatory disease in children.

69. Cavernous sinus thrombosis is often charactrized by, one is false:
    A. Rapid progression of the Proptosis
    B. Development of neurological signs
    C. Meningitis
    D. Lumbar puncture may show chronic inflammatory cells.

70. Which of the following is NOT a known cause of pulsatile proptosis?
    A. Neurofibromatosis type 1
    B. Orbital roof fracture
    C. Orbital meningoencephalocele
    D. Thyroid-associated orbitopathy.

71. The most common neoplasm of the lacrimal gland is:
    A. Lymphoproliferative disorders
    B. Adenoid cystic carcinoma
    C. Pleomorphic adenoma
    D. Malignant mixed tumour.

72. With regards to vascular tumours of the eyelids and orbit, one of the following is TRUE:
    A. Cavernous haemangioma causes gradual myopic shift
    B. Capillary hemagioma blanches with pressure
    C. Orbital varix causes proptosis at rest which is reduced by Valsalva manoeuvre
    D. Dural-cavernous fistula has a high blood-flow rate.

73. A high flow carotid cavernous fistula in a young man is likely to be due to:
    A. Congenital arteriovenous malformation
    B. Head trauma

C. Post radiation
D. Severe vasculitis.

74. Regarding optic nerve glioma one of the following statements is true:
    A. Predominantly seen in adults
    B. 90% associated with neurofibromatosis
    C. MRI can show cystic degeneration
    D. Expands within the optic nerve with no dural expansion.

75. 45 years old diabetic presented with one day history of right upper lid swelling, examination reveals normal visual acuity with prominent upper lid swelling, mild restriction of adduction and elevation with 2mm proptosis, the step that can be deferred to later would be:
    A. Admission and ordering of CT orbits
    B. Starting IV antibiotics
    C. Blood cultures
    D. Orthoptic evaluation of III nerve palsy.

76. The least possible complication of orbital cellulitis is:
    A. Ethmoidal sinusitis
    B. Cavernous sinus thrombosis
    C. Brain abscess
    D. Neurotrophic keratitis.

77. One of the followings is not a surgical space of the orbit
    A. The Extraconal surgical space
    B. The Subperiosteal space
    C. The supra-arachnoid space
    D. The episcleral surgical space.

78. Meningioma of the optic nerve is characterized by the following Except:
    A. Typically compresses the junction of chiasm with optic nerve
    B. Early visual field affection
    C. May cause loss of smell
    D. Early limitation of eye movement.

79. The majority of orbital lymphomas are:
    A. Polyclonal proliferation
    B. T-cell tumors
    C. Well differentiated
    D. Bilateral on presentation.

80. Pain and perineural invasion are associated with;
    A. Rhabdomyosarcoma
    B. Adenoid cystic carcinoma of the lacrimal gland

C. Esthisioneuroblastoma

D. Optic sheath meningioma.

81. Corticosteroids are used in treatment of all except;

    A. Orbital lymphoma

    B. Orbital mucocele

    C. Non specific orbital inflammation

    D. Wegener's granulomatosis.

82. What is the optimal imaging technique for a posterior optic nerve glioma?

    A. Plain X-ray films

    B. Computerized tomography

    C. Magnetic resonance imaging

    D. Ultrasound.

83. A patient with an optic-nerve sheath meningioma confined to the orbit has visual acuity of 20/30. What would be the best treatment at this stage?

    A. Radiation therapy

    B. Systemic steroid therapy

    C. Chemotherapy

    D. Observation.

84. In management of dermoid cysts of the orbit the most important to be considered is:

    A. Filling in any bony defects with bone substitute

    B. Removal of all cyst wall and cyst content

    C. All dermoids even if asymptomatic should be removed as early as possible.

    D. Deffering surgery till age 18 to avoid bony deformity.

85. Regarding dermoid cysts;

    A. Contain no dermal appendages

    B. Preseptal orbital dermoids are most commonly found in the medial upper eye lid

    C. Are lined by keratinizing epidermis

    D. Are always fixed to periosteum.

86. Regarding non specific orbital inflammation, which is false;

    A. It is a diagnosis of exclusion

    B. It should be differentiated from thyroid eye disease

C. Rapid reduction of systemic steroids may cause recurrence of inflammatory signs and symptoms

D. It is usually bilateral in adults.

87. Capillary hemangioma

    A. Enlarges dramatically during second year of life

    B. More common in the medial upper eyelid

    C. All should be treated as early as possible

    D. Seclerosing solution is highly recommended.

88. Orbital computed tomography scanning of a patient with a dural cavernous sinus fistula is likely to show enlargement of which one of the following blood vessels?

    A. Central retinal vein

    B. Pteregopalatine venous plexus

    C. Superior ophthalmic vein

    D. Inferior ophthalmic vein.

89. A pink-colored mass in the conjunctival fornix which appears as a salmon patch is typical for;

    A. Systemic lupus erythematouses

    B. Orbital lymphoma

    C. Lymphangioma

    D. Xanthogranuloma.

90. Orbital lymphoma is most commonly located in;

    A. The extra ocular muscles

    B. Retro orbital fat

    C. Lacrimal fossa

    D. Orbital apex.

91. Subperiosteal abscess of the orbit in adults is more likely than in children to;

    A. Drain spontaneously

    B. Respond to single antibiotic therapy

    C. Be Polymicrobial

    D. Arise from ethmoidal sinus.

92. Compared to CT scanning, MRI provide better;

    A. View of bone and calcium

    B. View of orbital apex and orbito-cranial junction

C. Elimination of motion artifact

D. Safety to patient with prosthetic implants.

93. A healthy 6 years old child presents with proptosis of the left eye, family phtographs reveal same prominence of the eye for the past year. One week prior to presentation the child had seizures. Fundus examination reveals choroidal folds in the left eye, which one of the following diagnostic test is least useful to be done;

A. Orbital ultrasound

B. MRI

C. Fluorescen angiography

D. CT scan.

94. On a T2 weighted MRI, which would appear hyperintense?

A. Fat

B. Blood in the carotid

C. Bone

D. Vitreous.

95. Which structure and its bony framework are paired INCORRECTLY?

A. Lacrimal sac fossa—lacrimal and maxillary bones

B. Optic canal—greater and lesser wings of the sphenoid bone

C. Inferior orbital fissure—maxilla, zygomtic bone, palatine bone, and greater wing of the sphenoid bone

D. Anterior and posterior ethmoidal foramen—ethmoid and frontal bones.

96. Which one of the following is the most common primary malignancy of the orbit in children?

A. Neuroblasroma

B. Rhabdomyosarcoma

C. Ewing's sarcoma

D. None of the above.

97. The following is TRUE about the superior ophthalmic vein:

A. It is the main venous channel of the orbit

B. It is formed by the union between the facial vein and the temporal vein

C. It passes backward in the orbit between the levator and the superior rectus muscle

D. It does not receives the central retinal vein.

98. The most common predisposing factor of orbital cellulitis is:

A. Dacryocystitis

B. Dental infection

C. Sinusitis

D. Trauma.

99. Limitation of ocular motility occurs in all except

A. Orbital margin fracture

B. Cavernous sinus thrombosis

C. Orbital cellulitis

D. Thyroid orbitopathy.

100. In orbital cystic lesions only one of the following statements is true;

A. Dermoid cyst is a hamartoma

B. Deep dermoid cysts typically present in infancy

C. Frontal mucocele may invade the orbit

D. Posterior encephalocele is characterized by pulsating proptosis and a bruit.

101. Medial wall of the orbit is formed by all except:

A. Ethmoid bone

B. Sphenoid bone

C. Frontal bone

D. Lacrimal bone.

102. Site of entry of inferior division of oculomotor nerve into the orbit is:

A. Inferior orbital fissure

B. Superior orbital fissure

C. Foramen lacerum

D. Foramen rotundum.

103. Structures passing through superior orbital fissure include all except:

A. II nd cranial nerve

B. III rd cranial nerve

C. IV th cranial nerve

D. VI th cranial nerve.

104. Purulent inflammation of the tissues of the orbit is called:

A. Orbital cellulitis

B. Endophthalmitis

C. Panophthalmitis

D. Dacryocystitis.

105. Which of the following conditions causes pseudoproptosis?

A. Hyperthyroidism

B. Orbital pseudotumour

C. High myopia

D. Optic nerve glioma.

106. Most common cause of unilateral proptosis in adults:

A. Thyroid ophthalmopathy

B. Rhabdomyosarcoma

C. Orbital cellulitis

D. Orbital blow out fracture.

107. Most common cause of unilateral proptosis in all age groups:

A. Thyrotoxicosis

B. Retinoblastoma

C. Intraocular haemorrhage

D. Raised lOP.

108. Most common cause of bilateral proptosis in children:

A. Rhabdomyosarcoma

B. Lymphoma

C. Retinoblastoma

D. Neuroblastoma.

109. A 45 years old female presents with unilateral mild axial proptosis. There is no redness or pain. Investigation of choice is:

A. T3 and T4 to rule out thyrotoxicosis

B. CT scan to rule out meningioma

C. Doppler to rule out haemangioma

D. USG to rule out orbital pseudotumour.

110. Infection from the dangerous area of the face spreads to the cavernous sinus via which of the following veins?

A. Maxillary veins

B. Retromandibular veins

C. Superficial temporal vein

D. Ophthalmic veins.

111. Paralysis of 3rd, 4th and 6th cranial nerves with involvement of ophthalmic division of the 5th cranial nerve localizes the lesion to:

A. Cavernous sinus

B. Apex of the orbit

C. Brainstem

D. Base of the skull.

112. A 19 years old young girl with previous history of repeated pain over medial canthus and chronic use of nasal decongestants presented with abrupt onset of fever and chills and rigors, diplopia on lateral gaze, moderate proptosis and chemosis. On examination, optic disc is congested. Most likely diagnosis is:

A. Cavernous sinus thrombosis

B. Orbital cellulitis

C. Acute ethmoidal sinusitis

D. Orbital apex syndrome.

113. All of the following could result from infection of the right cavernous sinus except:

A. Constricted pupil in response to light

B. Engorgement of retinal veins seen on ophthalmological examination

C. Ptosis of right eyelid

D. Right ophthalmoplegia.

114. A retrobulbar intraconal mass with well defined capsule presenting with slowly progressive proptosis in the 2nd to 4th decade is most likely:

A. Capillary haemangioma

B. Cavernous haemangioma

C. Lymphangioma

D. Haemangiopericytoma.

115. A patient presents with unilateral proptosis which is compressible and increases on bending forward. No thrill or bruit is present. MRI shows retrobulbar mass with enhancement. The likely diagnosis is:

A. A V malformation

B. Orbital varix

C. Orbital encephalocoele

D. Neurofibromatosis.

116. An 8-year-old boy presents with proptosis in the left eye for 3 months. CT scan reveals intraorbital extraconal mass lesion. Biopsy shows embryonal rhabdomyosarcoma. Metastatic workup is normal. The standard line of management is:

A. Chemotherapy

B. Wide local excision

C. Chemotherapy and radiotherapy

D. Enucleation.

117. In which side is the globe displaced in lacrimal gland tumour?
    A. Superior
    B. Inferonasal
    C. Inferotemporal
    D. Nasal.

118. Most common type of optic nerve glioma is:
    A. Gemiocytic
    B. Fibrous
    C. Protoplasmic
    D. Pilocytic.

119. Optic nerve glioma is associated with:
    A. Neurofibromatosis I
    B. Neurofibromatosis II
    C. Von Hippel Lindau disease
    D. Sturge Weber syndrome.

120. All of the following types of lymphoma may be seen in the orbit except:
    A. Non-Hodgkin's lymphoma, mixed lymphocytic and histiocytic
    B. Non-Hodgkin's lymphoma, poorly differentiated
    C. Burkitt's lymphoma
    D. Hodgkin's lymphoma.

121. The most common benign orbital tumor in children is:
    A. Capillary Hemangioma
    B. Dermoid cyst
    C. Lymphangioma
    D. Glioma.

122. The most common primary malignant orbital tumor in children is:
    A. Leukemia
    B. Rhabdomyosarcoma
    C. Neuroblastoma
    D. Lymphoma.

123. The most common orbital malignant tumor in adults is:
    A. Lymphoma
    B. Metastasis
    C. Lacrimal gland tumors
    D. Invasion from choroidal malignant melanoma.

124. The most common variety of Rhabdomyosarcoma is:
    A. Alveolar
    B. Pleomorphic
    C. Embryonal
    D. Mixed cellularity.

125. The least common variety of Rhabdomyosarcoma is:
    A. Alveolar
    B. Pleomorphic
    C. Embryonal
    D. Mixed cellularity.

126. The variety of Rhabdomyosarcoma with the best prognosis is:
    A. Alveolar
    B. Pleomorphic
    C. Embryonal
    D. Mixed cellularity.

127. The variety of Rhabdomyosarcoma with the worst prognosis is:
    A. Alveolar
    B. Pleomorphic
    C. Embryonal
    D. Mixed cellularity.

128. Chocolate cyst is due to bleeding in a
    A. Capillary hemangioma
    B. Cavernous hemangioma
    C. Lymphangioma
    D. Orbital varix.

129. Exentration is indicated in all the following conditions, except:
    A. Eyelid sebaceous carcinoma with deep orbital invasion
    B. Primary orbital rhabdomyosarcoma
    C. Extraocular extension of melanoma without systemic metastasis
    D. Orbital phycomycosis.

130. The following clinical features are characteristic of adenoid cystic carcinoma of the lacrimal gland except:
    A. Occurrence in old age group
    B. Rapid progression over weeks to months
    C. Presence of bone erosion
    D. Hypesthesia in the temporal region.

131. All of the following clinical features are characteristic of lymphoid tumors of the lacrimal gland, except:
    A. Bony remodeling
    B. Absence of globe ptosis
    C. More anterior location
    D. Soft to palpation.

132. The following disorders typically produces downward and lateral displacement of the globe?
    A. Malignant mixed tumor of the lacrimal gland
    B. Squamous cell carcinoma of the maxillary sinus
    C. Frontal sinus mucocele
    D. Optic nerve sheath meningioma.
133. All of the following disorders typically present with a rapid onset, except
    A. Ruptured dermoid cyst
    B. Benign mixed tumor of the lacrimal gland
    C. Rhabdomyosarcoma
    D. Orbital cellulitis.
134. An orbital meningocele usually presents in the:
    A. Supraorbital notch
    B. Lateral canthus
    C. Lacrimal gland fossa
    D. Medial canthus.
135. A traumatic carotid cavernous fistula results in all of the following, except
    A. Elevated orbital arterial pressure
    B. Audible bruit
    C. Tortous conjunctival vessels extending to the limbus
    D. Extraocular muscle enlargement.
136. The most common orbital or eyelid finding in the craniosynostosis syndromes is
    A. Ankyloblepharon
    B. Ptosis
    C. Exotropia
    D. Hypertelorism and proptosis.
137. Which of the following is true of breast cancer metastatic to the orbit?
    A. The majority of orbital metastases in women originate from breast cancer
    B. Patients will likely benefit from hormone therapy
    C. Bone metastasis is more common than extraocular muscle involvement
    D. Enophthalmos is more common than proptosis.
138. Which of the following can be associated with multiple large capillary hemangiomas?
    A. Thrombocytosis
    B. Thrombocytopenia
    C. Leukocytosis
    D. Leukocytopenia.
139. A patient with suspected orbital cellulitis develops loss of ocular motility with intact vision. The most likely diagnosis is
    A. Cavernous sinus thrombosis
    B. Orbital compartment syndrome
    C. Meningitis secondary to orbital cellulitis
    D. Orbital apex syndrome.
140. Enophthalmos can occur in all of the following except
    A. Silent sinus syndrome
    B. Orbital varix
    C. Medial wall orbital fracture
    D. Malar hypoplasia.
141. Nevus flammeus occurs in:
    A. Neurofibromatosis
    B. Treacher Collins' syndrome
    C. Von Hippel's disease
    D. Sturge-Weber syndrome.
142. Most periocular capillary hemangiomas manifest by
    A. 4 to 8 weeks of age
    B. 6 to 8 months of age
    C. 12 to 18 months of age
    D. 3 to 4 years of age.
143. Most capillary hemangiomas reach their peak size at:
    A. 2 to 3 months
    B. 9 to 12 months
    C. 18 to 24 months
    D. 3 to 5 years.
144. A characteristic feature distinguishing between nevus flammeus and capillary hemangioma is
    A. Lesion color
    B. Presence or absence of blanching with pressure
    C. Area of skin affected
    D. Extent of skin thickening.
145. Regarding orbital rhabdomyosarcoma, which is incorrect?
    A. Metastatic workup includes lumbar puncture and bone marrow biopsy
    B. Alveolar rhabdomyosarcoma, occurs most frequently in the superior orbit

C. Electron microscopic studies may be used in facilitating the diagnosis, as cross-striations are more apparent on electron microscopy

D. The embryonal pattern is the most common pathologic variant, accounting for more than 80% of total cases.

146. A patient with known neurofibromatosis presents with pulsating proptosis of long duration. CT scan of the orbit will most likely reveal
   A. Orbital neurofibroma
   B. Abnormality of the sphenoid bone
   C. Optic nerve glioma
   D. Carotid-cavernous fistula.

147. A patient with diabetes mellitus presenting with orbital cellulitis requires immediate:
   A. Complete blood count
   B. Oral temperature
   C. Blood glucose measurement
   D. Careful ear, nose, and throat evaluation.

148. Compared with adults, all of the following findings are more common in pediatric idiopathic orbital inflammation (orbital pseudotumor), except
   A. Uveitis
   B. Optic disc edema
   C. Unilateral presentation
   D. Eosinophilia.

149. All of the following disorders may be associated with a clinical presentation indistinguishable from typical inflammatory orbital pseudotumor, except
   A. Wegener's granulomatosis
   B. Churg-Strauss syndrome
   C. Sarcoidosis
   D. Polyarteritis nodosa.

150. A 3-year-old boy presents with a painless lesion of the lateral left upper eyelid and brow. The lesion is smooth and fixed to the underlying bone. Which of the following statements is true:
   A. An eyelid crease incision usually does not provide sufficient exposure
   B. The lesion is classified as a hamartoma
   C. The condition may occur along the superomedial orbital rim

D. The lesion is lined by nonkeratinizing squamous epithelium with dermal appendages.

151. A 45-year-old woman presents with an encapsulated well-circumscribed retrobulbar mass. All of the following are potential diagnoses, except
   A. Neurilemoma
   B. Hemangiopericytoma
   C. Lymphangioma
   D. Fibrous histiocytoma.

152. Which one of the following regarding dermoid and epidermoid cysts is false?
   A. They share a common pathophysiology
   B. The key distinguishing feature between the two is the nature of the wall of the cystic cavity
   C. In adults, nearly all of these lesions are anterior to the orbital septum
   D. Superficial cysts present more often during childhood.

153. A patient presents with slowly progressive proptosis of the right eye. Excisional biopsy confirms large cavernous spaces containing erythrocytes. All of the following may be seen in this condition, except
   A. Accelerated growth of the lesion in a pregnant patient
   B. Anterior displacement of the far point plane of the eye
   C. More than one type of optic neuropathy
   D. Radiodense phleboliths present on CT scan tmagmg.

154. What is the expected reflectivity on A-scan ultrasonography of the capsule of cavernous hemangioma?
   A. None
   B. Low
   C. Medium
   D. High.

155. A 2-year-old child presents with bilateral proptosis. Which of the following is the least likely diagnosis?
   A. Metastatic neuroblastoma
   B. Leukemia
   C. Capillary hemangioma
   D. Orbital pseudotumor.

156. The most common sinus lesion that invades the orbit is the
    A. Osteoma
    B. Inverted papilloma
    C. Mucocele
    D. Squamous cell carcinoma.

157. What is the treatment of choice for a patient with an optic nerve sheath meningioma confined to the orbit and with progressive visual loss?
    A. Observation
    B. Surgical excision
    C. Chemotherapy
    D. Radiation therapy.

158. An 86-year-old patient presents with left eye proptosis, diplopia, and a subconjunctival salmon patch lesion. Which of the following is the most appropriate next step?
    A. Biopsy
    B. B-scan ultrasonography
    C. Corticosteroids
    D. Orbital imaging.

159. A 7-year-old boy presents with a 3-day history of progressive proptosis, injection, and pain of the left eye. He is systemically well with normal temperature. White blood cell count is normal, and orbital CT scanning reveals superonasal orbital infiltration with bony erosion. The most likely diagnosis at this point is
    A. Frontal sinus mucocele
    B. Rhabdomyosarcoma
    C. Bacterial orbital cellulitis
    D. Optic nerve glioma.

160. Which one of the following histiocytic disorders is most likely to involve orbital bone?
    A. Sinus histiocytosis
    B. Hand-Schtiller-Christian disease
    C. Letterer-Siwe disease
    D. Eosinophilic granuloma.

161. Which of the following is one of the most common mesenchymal tumor of the orbit?
    A. Hemangiopericytoma
    B. Fibrous histiocytoma
    C. Osteogenic sarcoma
    D. Ossifying fibroma.

162. The most common site of a primary tumor metastatic to the orbit in men is
    A. Lung
    B. Colon
    C. Prostate
    D. Melanoma.

163. In a 10 years old patient with optic nerve glioma, which one of the following clinical features would be considered inconsistent with the diagnosis?
    A. Unilaterality
    B. Insidious onset
    C. Afferent pupillary defect
    D. Pain.

164. Which of the following answers would be the best treatment option for a localized orbital lymphoproliferative lesion?
    A. Radiation and systemic corticosteroids
    B. Radiation therapy alone
    C. Surgical excision combined with chemotherapy
    D. Surgical excision combined with radiation.

165. Hyperostotic lesions of the orbit can occur in all, except
    A. Metastatic prostate carcinoma
    B. Sphenoid wing meningioma
    C. Fibrous dysplasia
    D. Metastatic melanoma.

166. An 11-year-old patient presents with acute, unilateral, left-sided periocular pain, proptosis, and double vision. Which condition would *not* be included in the differential diagnosis?
    A. Cavernous hemangioma
    B. Sinusitis with orbital abscess
    C. Traumatic retrobulbar hemorrhage
    D. Orbital lymphangioma.

167. Twenty-four hours later (and without any treatment), the pain has resolved. Periocular ecchymosis has developed, and the double vision has stabilized. The most likely diagnosis based on the clinical history:
    A. Rhabdomyosarcoma
    B. Capillary hemangioma
    C. Orbital abscess
    D. Lymphangioma.

168. If the patient was losing vision because of this process, you would consider:
    A. Open surgery to excise the lesion in its entirety
    B. CT-directed drainage of the encysted blood
    C. Injection of sclerosing agents
    D. Radiotherapy.

169. This disease process is an example of:
    A. The most common cause of proptosis in children
    B. The most common primary orbital malignancy in children
    C. A tumor that may enlarge with upper respiratory infections
    D. An orbital vascular lesion that will involute after intralesional corticosteroids.

170. In orbital infectious disease:
    A. The presence of a subperiosteal collection of fluid is an indication for surgery
    B. The onset of decreased vision and an afferent pupillary defect in the presence of an orbital abscess is an indication for surgery
    C. Proptosis and limitation of motility differentiate an orbital abscess from orbital cellulitis
    D. The maxillary sinus is the most common sinus involved when orbital cellulitis occurs as a result of sinusitis.

171. A 6 years old patient has a 2-week history of rapidly progressing superonasal mass that does not affect vision. Examination shows proptosis pushing the eye down and out. The best management includes all of the following except:
    A. CT scan
    B. Anterior orbitotomy with biopsy
    C. MRI scan
    D. Observation.

172. A 48 years old female who is otherwise healthy has a 2 years old slowly progressing painless proptosis with normal vision. what is the most likely diagnosis?
    A. Optic nerve glioma
    B. Cavernous hemangioma
    C. Metastatic breast cancer

    D. Benign mixed cell tumor of the lacrimal gland.

173. The orbital ultrasound would show:
    A. Tissue of homogenous character
    B. High internal reflectivity
    C. B scan identifying tumor in the anterior inferior orbit
    D. Low amplitude internal echoes.

174. The natural history of such lesion is:
    A. Slow growth over several years
    B. Erosion of surrounding bony structure
    C. Displacement of the globe downward and medially
    D. Potential for malignant conversion of the presently benign lesion.

175. Surgical removal of the lesion would best be approached by:
    A. A lateral orbitotomy with en bloc removal of the mass
    B. Incisional biopsy followed by radiation or chemotherapy
    C. An anterior approach through the inferior fornix
    D. A medial orbitotomy with reflection of the medial rectus muscle.
    A 60-years-old woman presents with painless swelling of the lacrimal gland and anterior orbit for 2 months. There is no significant history.

176. What is the most likely diagnosis?
    A. Primary lacrimal gland lymphoma
    B. Pleomorphic adenoma
    C. Adenoid cystic carcinoma
    D. Malignant pleomorphic adenoma.

177. What is the most accurate description of the pathology specimen taken from this lesion?
    A. Spindle cells with both ductal epithelium and a mixed stromal pattern
    B. "Swiss cheese" pattern-hyperchromatic small cells proliferating around nerves
    C. Ductal epithelium in a tubular formation with malignant degeneration
    D. Mixture of both B and T cells, with predominance of B cells.

178. The most common cause of bilateral exophthalmos in adults is:
    A. Cavernous hemangioma

B. Pseudotumor

C. Thyroid-related orbitopathy

D. Metastatic disease.

179. What is the most common cause of unilateral childhood exophthalmos?

A. Capillary hemangioma

B. Thyroid-related orbitopathy

C. Orbital hemorrhage

D. Orbital cellulitis.

180. Predisposing conditions for mucormycosis include:

A. Diabetes

B. Renal disease

C. Dehydration

D. All of the above.

181. Proper treatment of orbital mucormycosis includes all of the following except:

A. Stabilizing the underlying disease process

B. Debridement of all devitalized tissue, including exenteration if necessary

C. Amphotericin B for 6 weeks

D. Radiation to the orbit.

182. Indications for closure of carotid cavernous sinus fistulas does not include which of the following?

A. Ophthalmoplegia

B. Severe headache

C. Persistent bruit

D. Progressive proptosis.

183. Which of the following sequelae of a carotid cavernous sinus fistula is the most common cause of visual disability?

A. Strabismus

B. Proptosis with corneal exposure

C. Spontaneous choroidal detachment

D. Elevated intraocular pressure with progressive optic nerve damage.

184. A non-painful, well-circumscribed homogenous spherical mass in the inferior orbit that moderately enhances with contrast in an otherwise healthy patient who complains of diplopia is best treated by:

A. Chemotherapy

B. Radiation therapy

C. Surgical excision

D. Observation.

185. A 61-year-old patient, with a chronic sinus problem presents with a 1-week history of redness and pain of the right eye. His visual acuity is 20/20. His right upper eyelid is swollen. The right conjunctiva is injected with dilated episcleral vessels inferiorly. The underlying sclera appears inflamed. His ocular motility is limited, and there is 2 mm of proptosis. A CT scan shows a diffuse infiltrate in the right inferior orbit. There is also thickening of the left nasal mucosa. Which of the following tests would be most beneficial in diagnosing this patient's condition?

A. Serum c-ANCA (antineutrophil cytoplasmic antibodies)

B. Serum p-ANCA (antineutrophil cytoplasmic antibodies)

C. Serum ESR (erythrocyte sedimentation rate) and C-reactive protein

D. Conjunctival culture for bacterial and viral pathogens.

186. A 50-year-old patient presents with a 4-day history of right eyelid swelling, conjunctival injection, and pain and double vision. Visual acuity is normal. There is normal pupillary reactions. There is a small abduction deficit 0D. The right upper eyelid is erythematous and swollen. The conjunctiva is injected and chemotic. Deeper episcleral vessels are injected. The cornea is clear and the anterior chamber is quiet. The left eye is normal. Fundus examination is normal. There is 2 mm of proptosis 0D. CT scan of the orbits shows diffuse soft tissue infiltrate involving the anterior portion of the right orbit. The nasal mucosa appears thickened on the left side. The patient has no fever, and laboratory studies are normal with no evidence of diabetes. After 7 days on oral corticosteroids, the patient shows moderate improvement. He has less pain, and redness and eyelid swelling have decreased. However, the proptosis and diplopia are unchanged. Which of the following is the most appropriate next step?

A. Start intravenous corticosteroids

B. Continue the present treatment for 1 more week

C. Remove tissue from the right orbit for biopsy

D. Repeat the CT scan of the orbits.

187. A 2-year-old girl has left lower eyelid ecchymosis. There is 3 mm of proptosis of the left eye. Her medical history is significant for treatment of some unknown tumor. Which of the following childhood tumors is the most likely diagnosis?
    A. Rhabdomyosarcoma
    B. Retinoblastoma
    C. Neuroblastoma
    D. Leukemia.

188. A 56-year-old man complains of an aching sensation around his left eye for 6 weeks. The discomfort increases on upgaze. One week ago, he noted blurred vision in the left eye and a low-grade fever. His visual acuity is 20/20 OD and 20/40 OS. The patient has 3 mm of proptosis in the left eye and mild erythema and tenderness around the left eyelid. What is the most helpful diagnostic test for this patient?
    A. CT scan of the orbits
    B. Complete blood count
    C. Thyroid function tests
    D. Skull films.

189. Which of the following orbital diseases is least likely to improve with corticosteroids?
    A. Orbital mucocele
    B. Thyroid-related orbitopathy
    C. Orbital pseudotumor
    D. Orbital lymphoma.

190. Which of the following is not a potential advantage of MRI over CT scanning?
    A. MRI does not expose the patient to radiation
    B. MRI is unaffected by motion artifact
    C. MRI can generate high quality axial, coronal, and sagittal image without repositioning the patient
    D. MRI allows for better evaluation of lesions that extend from the orbit to the cranium.

191. Computerized tomography has demonstrated an orbital bone mass to have a "ground glass" appearance. What systemic involvement should be ruled out?
    A. Generalized muscle weakness
    B. Visceral cancer
    C. Thyroid disease
    D. Endocrine abnormality.

192. During routine examination of a patient's inferior cul-de-sac, a subconjunctival lympho-proliferative lesion is observed. The patient is unaware of this lesion and is reportedly in good health. The results of the remainder of the ocular examination are normal. A biopsy is done. What would the least useful test performed on this biopsy be?
    A. Permanent sections
    B. Culture and sensitivity
    C. Cell-surface markers
    D. Electron microscopy.

193. What is the best study to rule out organic orbital foreign bodies?
    A. Magnetic resonance imaging
    B. A dowsing rod
    C. Plain films
    D. Computerized tomography.

194. What is the study of choice for the evaluation of fractures in acute orbital trauma?
    A. Orbital ultrasound
    B. Computerized tomography
    C. Magnetic resonance imaging
    D. Nerve conduction.

195. The myositic form of idiopathic orbital inflammation is associated with which of the following conditions?
    A. Efficacy of systemic steroid therapy
    B. S-shaped deformity of the eyelid
    C. Fusiform enlargement of extraocular muscle involving the tendon
    D. Nodular enlargement of the extraocular muscle belly.

196. What is a common sign of a malignant lymphoproliferative lesion?
    A. Firm nodular anterior orbital mass
    B. Painful proptosis
    C. Vision loss
    D. Madarosis.

197. What is the optimal imaging technique for a posterior optic nerve glioma?
    A. Magnetic resonance imaging
    B. Plain X-ray films
    C. Computerized tomography
    D. Orbital ultrasound.

198. When diplopia develops in the setting of traumatic carotid cavernous fistula, what is the most likely pathophysiology?
    A. Compression of the fourth cranial nerve as it exits the brainstem
    B. Compression of the superior rectus muscle within the muscle cone
    C. Damage to the third cranial nerve from elevated intracranial pressure
    D. Compression of the sixth cranial nerve within the cavernous sinus.

199. What is the test of choice when considering treatment for a carotid cavernous fistula?
    A. Computed tomography
    B. Magnetic resonance imaging
    C. Conventional angiography
    D. Computed tomographic angiography.

200. What would you expect to find on computerized axial tomography (CT) of a dural sinus fistula?
    A. Extraocular muscle enlargement
    B. Phleboliths
    C. Enlargement of the internal carotid artery
    D. Orbital expansion with Valsalva maneuver.

201. For which orbital disease can increased orbital fat volume be a primary radiographic finding?
    A. Orbital myositis
    B. Thyroid orbitopathy
    C. Sarcoidosis
    D. Wegner's granulomatosis.

202. A 6-year-old presents with proptosis and inferior-lateral displacement of the globe. Imaging demonstrates clear sinuses and a large orbital mass. What step should be considered next?
    A. Prompt biopsy with possible frozen section diagnosis, bone marrow biopsy, and lumbar puncture

    B. Attempted aspiration of the mass with empiric antibiotics if aspiration is unsuccessful
    C. Discharge home on oral antibiotics
    D. Treat with intravenous antibiotics for 10 days and reevaluate.

203. What is the preferred management of hemangiopericytoma involving the orbit?
    A. Incisional biopsy followed by external radiation
    B. Intralesional steroid injection
    C. Observation
    D. Complete local excision.

204. A 35-year-old woman has decreased visual acuity in the right eye over 3 years. The visual acuity in the left eye is 20/20. Examination of the right eye shows visual acuity of 20/70, a right afferent pupillary defect, 3 mm axial proptosis and bilaterally normal optic discs. What is the most likely diagnosis?
    A. Adenoid cystic carcinoma of lacrimal gland
    B. Orbital lymphoma
    C. Optic nerve glioma
    D. Optic nerve sheath meningioma.

205. What tissue provides such a bright signal on a T1-weighted, magnetic resonance image (MRI) that it can obscure important structures?
    A. Bone
    B. Fat
    C. Vitreous
    D. Lens.

206. What pathologic finding is found in idiopathic orbital inflammation?
    A. Monoclonal hypercellular lymphoid proliferation
    B. Polyclonal hypercellular lymphoid proliferation
    C. Granulomatous cellular infiltrate
    D. Pleomorphic cellular infiltrate.

207. In a young child with a subperiosteal orbital abscess, in what location(s) would medical therapy be preferred to surgical drainage?
    A. Lateral orbit
    B. Orbital apex

C. Medial orbit

D. Superior orbit.

208. What is the prognosis of mucosal-associated lymphoid tissue (MALT) mass in the orbit?

   A. Orbital enlargement, metastasis in half of patients within 10 years

   B. Usually progresses to large-cell lymphoma

   C. Rapid orbital enlargement, metastasis in nearly all patients within 10 years

   D. Benign ocular and systemic morbidity.

209. A febrile 65-year-old diabetic has orbital cellulitis with severe edema, areas of gray skin discoloration and tissue necrosis. The sinuses are clear. What would be the preferred treatment?

   A. Amphotericin B

   B. Surgical debridement, broad-spectrum antibiotics, and probably ICU support

   C. System steroids

   D. Hyperbaric oxygen.

210. Regarding lymphangiomas, which is incorrect:

   A. Often appear at birth or during early childhood

   B. May cause proptosis after they hemorrhage

   C. Are connected to the orbital lymphatic system

   D. May enlarge with systemic viral illness.

211. Regarding juvenile xanthogranuloma (JXG), which is incorrect:

   A. Most commonly involves the skin of the head and neck

   B. May involve the iris, leading to spontaneous hyphema

   C. Is a benign histiocytic proliferation

   D. If intraocular, usually involutes with time.

212. Regarding metastatic tumors to the orbit, which is incorrect:

   A. Develop before diagnosis of the primary tumor in 30–60% of patients

   B. Reach the orbit by hematogenous spread

   C. In children are usually carcinomas

   D. Are often painful in men who have prostate cancer.

213. Regarding pleomorphic adenoma of the lacrimal gland (benign mixed cell tumor), which is incorrect:

   A. Occurs mainly in the palpebral lobe

   B. Represents 50% of epithelial lacrimal gland tumors

   C. Most commonly occurs in the second to fifth decades of life

   D. May be cystic and contain calcification.

214. Regarding adenoid cystic carcinoma of the lacrimal gland, which is incorrect:

   A. Is rarely painful

   B. Has a dismal prognosis, even with treatment

   C. May be seen at any age but is more common in the fourth decades of life

   D. Is the most common epithelial malignancy of the lacrimal gland.

215. Regarding fibrous dysplasia of the orbit, which is incorrect:

   A. May cause vision loss from compression of the optic nerve in the optic canal

   B. Usually is poly-ostotic

   C. Replaces normal bone with immature bone and osteoid

   D. Usually is progressive until the second or third decade of life.

216. Regarding rhabdomyosarcoma, which is incorrect:

   A. Requires immediate biopsy to confirm the diagnosis

   B. Is most commonly the embryonal form

   C. Involves a 5-year survival rate in 45% of affected individuals

   D. Is the most common soft tissue primary malignant mesenchymal orbital tumor in children.

217. Regarding plexiform neurofibroma, which is incorrect:

   A. Is the most common benign peripheral nerve tumor involving the eyelids and orbit

   B. Is characteristic of neurofibromatosis

   C. Is not invasive

   D. Has a propensity for sensory nerves.

218. Regarding neuroblastoma that is metastatic to the orbit, which is incorrect:
    A. First appears as an orbital mass in 8% of cases
    B. Is the second most common malignant orbital tumor of childhood
    C. Affects both orbits in 40% of children
    D. Rarely advances to orbital bones.

219. Regarding malignant orbital lymphoma, which is incorrect:
    A. Usually contains proliferated B cells
    B. Is bilateral in 75% of cases
    C. Is associated with systemic lymphoma in 40% of patients at the time of diagnosis
    D. Is treatable and has an excellent visual prognosis.

220. Regarding orbital dermoid cysts, which is incorrect:
    A. May be subtotally resected with good results
    B. May lie deep in the orbit
    C. Are lined with epithelium and filled with keratinized material
    D. Represent 25% of all orbital and lid masses.

221. Diagnostic criteria for IgG4 related orbitopathy includes all except:
    A. Characteristic swelling in the orbit
    B. Elevated serum IgG4
    C. Histopathological evidence of lymphocytic proliferation
    D. Excellent response to steroid treatment.

222. The biologic response modifier, rituximab, binds to which of the following targets?
    A. CDlla
    B. CD20
    C. CD25
    D. TNF-a.

223. Langerhans cell histiocytosis include all except:
    A. Eosinophilic granuloma
    B. Kassabach–Merritt syndrome
    C. Hand-Schuller–Christian disease
    D. Letterer–Siwe disease.

224. Which of the following statements about rhabdomyosarcoma is correct?
    A. The most common extracranial solid childhood tumour
    B. Embryonal and alveolar subtypes have distinct genetic alterations that may play in the pathogenesis of the tumors
    C. Orbital tumours are more likely to have alveolar histologic subtype
    D. Orbital tumours commonly present with ophthalmoplegia.

225. Which of the following statements about neurofibromatosis type 1 is correct?
    A. More than 50% of patients with NF1 have learning difficulties
    B. Lab tests are useful in the diagnosis of NF1
    C. Lisch nodules are the most characteristic feature in children over six years of age
    D. Choroidal hamartomas are well-defined, elevated lesions found in the midperiphery of the retina.

226. Which of the following signs would you expect to see in a patient presenting with a suspected direct carotico-cavernous fistula (CCF) after an injury but not in a spontaneous indirect CCF?
    A. Acute painful proptosis
    B. Cranial bruit
    C. Dilated episcleral vessels
    D. Raised intraocular pressure (lOP).

227. A 4-year-old child presents as an emergency with a 2-day history of unilateral periocular swelling, redness, and proptosis. Which of the following is NOT an essential emergency investigation?
    A. Full blood count
    B. Temperature
    C. Plain film X-ray face
    D. Weight.

228. During a surgical decompression for acute compressive optic neuropathy which of the paranasal sinuses will NOT be entered?
    A. Ethmoid
    B. Frontal
    C. Maxillary
    D. Sphenoid.

229. A 40-year-old female presents with a 3-month history of painful swelling in the superotemporal quadrant of the left orbit. She undergoes an incision biopsy which demonstrates glandular tubules with lumina, excess basement membrane and mucin, and islands of anaplastic cells without squamous differentiation. Which of the following is the most likely diagnosis?
   A. Adenoid cystic carcinoma
   B. Dacryoadenitis
   C. Pleomorphic adenoma
   D. Sarcoidosis.

230. In a patient with an isolated lacrimal gland mass, what test would be the most sensitive to differentiate between lymphoma and orbital inflammatory disease (OID)?
   A. Contrast enhanced MRI
   B. Orbital biopsy
   C. Serum LDH
   D. Steroid response.

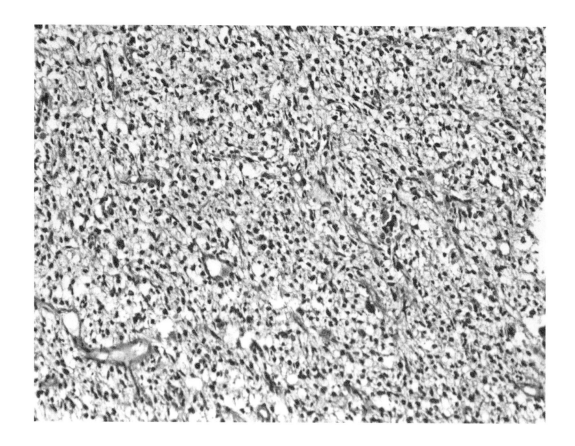

231. The above histopathological figures points to the diagnosis of which type of rhabdomyosarcoma:
   A. Alveolar
   B. Embryonal
   C. Mixed
   D. Pleomorphic.

Answer for the Orbit

30	C	60	C	90	C	120	D
121	B	151	C	181	D	211	D
122	B	152	C	182	C	212	C
123	A	153	B	183	A	213	A
124	C	154	D	184	C	214	A
125	B	155	C	185	A	215	B
126	B	156	C	186	C	216	C
127	A	157	D	187	C	217	C
128	C	158	D	188	A	218	D
129	B	159	B	189	A	219	B
130	A	160	D	190	B	220	A
131	A	161	B	191	D	221	D
132	C	162	A	192	B	222	B
133	B	163	D	193	A	223	B
134	D	164	B	194	B	224	B
135	A	165	D	195	D	225	A
136	D	166	A	196	A	226	B
137	A	167	D	197	A	227	C
138	B	168	B	198	D	228	B
139	A	169	C	199	C	229	A
140	D	170	B	200	A	230	B
141	D	171	D	201	B	231	B
142	A	172	B	202	A		
143	B	173	B	203	D		
144	B	174	A	204	D		
145	B	175	A	205	B		
146	B	176	A	206	D		
147	D	177	D	207	C		
148	C	178	C	208	A		
149	C	179	D	209	B		
150	C	180	D	210	C		

1	B	31	B	61	C	91	C
2	C	32	A	62	D	92	B
3	B	33	B	63	B	93	C
4	A	34	B	64	B	94	A
5	B	35	B	65	B	95	C
6	B	36	D	66	C	96	B
7	D	37	B	67	A	97	A
8	B	38	C	68	D	98	B
9	C	39	A	69	D	99	A
10	D	40	C	70	D	100	C
11	C	41	D	71	A	101	C
12	C	42	A	72	B	102	B
13	C	43	C	73	B	103	A
14	D	44	D	74	C	104	A
15	B	45	A	75	D	105	C
16	B	46	A	76	A	106	A
17	B	47	D	77	C	107	A
18	B	48	B	78	D	108	D
19	C	49	D	79	C	109	A
20	C	50	B	80	B	110	D
21	D	51	A	81	B	111	A
22	C	52	C	82	C	112	A
23	C	53	C	83	D	113	A
24	B	54	D	84	B	114	B
25	D	55	A	85	C	115	B
26	C	56	D	86	D	116	C
27	B	57	D	87	B	117	B
28	A	58	B	88	C	118	D
29	A	59	D	89	B	119	A

Orbital Implants and Prosthesis

9

Essam A. El Toukhy

Eye Removal Surgery (enucleation or evisceration) is often considered as a lost battle in ophthalmology as there is no hope for restoring vision. The technique of eye removal is constantly evolving. Sufferers bears the stigma of disfigurement and some gets disturbed psychologically. One simple solution in most of these cases is to fit a custom-designed ocular prosthesis (or an artificial eye) that looks like a natural eye and can even move (to varied extent in different conditions). The psychological aspects of loss of an eye should always be addressed by the oculoplastic surgeon and the ocularist and patients may even need the help of a clinical psychologist particularly in children and young adults. Organizing meetings with the ocularist prior to eye removal surgery can be helpful in this regard.

The ideal socket is a centrally placed well covered implant of adequate size fabricated from an inert material. It should have deep unobstructed fornices with an inferior lid and fornix that can adequately support the prosthetic eye. The superior eyelid should be symmetrical with the normal eyelid, and finally prosthetic movement should approach the normal side.

Evisceration is a surgical procedure involving the surgical removal of the intraocular contents of the globe with or without keratectomy. It involves minimal disruption of the orbital contents with the best cosmetic result over enucleation. It is contraindicated in a patient who has a history of intraocular tumor. In a blind eye, a B scan ultrasound must be done to rule out an occult tumor. Expansion sclerotomies have improved the outcomes in eviscervation surgical technique. The procedure takes less time than enucleation surgery and can be done under general or monitored assisted anesthesia with minimal complications.

Evisceration from a practical point of view makes sense. Easy to perform, minimal complications and provides good motility. It is a surgical procedure in which the entire contents of the globe are removed through a corneal, limbal or scleral incision. The extraocular muscles are not detached from the sclera, and the optic nerve and its surrounding meninges are left undisturbed. Although the cornea was traditionally always removed, most surgeons now preserve it. In the event that expansions cannot house an adequate implant, the posterior sclera can be totally transected and an alloplastic sphere placed in the intraconal space.

General anesthesia is not usually needed, monitored attended local anesthesia is very effective. A retrobulbar block and frontal block anesthesia must be used for intraoperative and postoperative pain management due to postoperative discomfort and swelling.

E. A. El Toukhy (✉)
Oculoplasty Service, Cairo University, Cairo, Egypt
e-mail: eeltoukhy@yahoo.com

© The Author(s), under exclusive license to Springer Nature Switzerland AG 2021
E. A. El Toukhy (ed.), *Oculoplasty for Ophthalmologists*, https://doi.org/10.1007/978-3-030-68469-3_9

Surgeons performing enucleation must take into account movement of the prosthesis after surgery and the potential postoperative complications such as implant extrusion or socket contraction. The optimal size of the chosen sphere should be such that when it is placed within the orbit, the muscles can be tied over the implant without any tension.

Enucleation or evisceration can be performed without placement of an orbital implant, but this will result in suboptimal cosmetic outcome. An orbital implant replaces the lost volume in eviscerated or enucleated globe, impart motility to the prosthesis, supports surrounding structures and thus maintain cosmetic symmetry with the fellow eye.

A large number of implants are available today. An ideal implant is the one which fulfills the following criteria:

- Integration with orbital tissues
- Biocompatible: It should not cause any allergic or inflammatory reaction or rejection
- Non-biodegradable
- Free from complications like infection, extrusion and migration
- Adequate volume replacement
- Adequate support for prosthesis
- Allow maximum motility with prosthesis
- Stimulate orbital growth
- Readily available, inexpensive and easy to use/implant.

It is crucial to place an optimum size implant. Smaller implants tend to migrate and does not solve the purpose of adequate volume replacement. Larger implant interferes with the aesthetics and tension on the conjunctival wound that could result in wound gap and implant extrusion. Ideally, 65–70% of the volume should be replaced by implant and remaining 30–35% with the prosthesis. The recent introduction of non-spherical (conical or egg-shaped) implants has made it possible to increase the volume of the implant without the need to increase its anterior curvature.

An algorithm was developed to assess the optimal orbital implant size when performing a preoperative A-scan of the fellow eye. The use of A-scan ultrasonography of the fellow healthy eye to provide a tool for correct orbital implant size to replace 80% of the volume removed at enucleation. This method allows a gap in the anterior socket for an ocular prosthetic volume of 2 mL when the orbital implant is placed deep in the intraconal space. The algorithm divides the preoperative A-scan values into hyperopes and emmetropes/myopes for final orbital implant size calculations. The algorithm can be used to preoperatively calculate the proper orbital implant size for both adults and children undergoing enucleation or evisceration procedures.

A major focus of research and development in the last couple of decades is the newer materials for orbital implant and improvement in prosthesis motility. Porous materials are currently preferred primarily because of vascularization and integration that occur. These implants are less likely to migrate than silicone or PMMA implants and are associated with better prosthesis motility especially when coupled with a peg. However, hydroxyapatite and porous polyethylene are significantly more expensive and are associated with higher rates of exposure than traditional non integrated implants. Wrapping or "capping" these implants appears to reduce the exposure rate to acceptable levels. Implant size is crucial and should be customized. Implant motility is primarily determined by the attachment of extraocular muscles to the implant. Placement of wrapped silicone or PMMA implant with extraocular muscle attachment provides excellent results in patients who do not wish to consider a motility peg placement. Porous implants should be used in patients who are keen on further enhanced motility.

Hydroxyapatite-First introduced by Perry in 1985, the implant material is made of a complex calcium phosphate salt normally found in human mineralized bone and derived from living corals found deep in the oceans. It is biocompatible, non-biodegradable, non-toxic and non-allergenic. The porous matrix is infiltrated by the orbital fibrovascular tissue. Vascularisation of the implant can be assessed radiographically with contrast enhanced Magnetic Resonance Imaging (MRI) with surface coil. Implants with grade 3 or 4 vascularisation (equal to or greater than the orbital rim) are considered as adequately vascularized. The assessment of vascularization is essential before drilling a hole for pegging to identify the central avascular zone. Implants with more than 75% vascularization also tend to bleed more during drilling. The extent of vascularization can be influenced by the pore structure and orientation of the pores. Poor vascularization can lead to implant extrusion. The rough surface of the porous implants can cause erosion of the conjunctiva and Tenon's and ultimately cause exposure of the implant. This can be prevented by wrapping the implant with appropriate materials.

Porous polyethylene implants are normally well tolerated in the orbital soft tissue. They are easier to implant because they have a smoother surface than HA implants, and potentially cause less irritation of the overlying conjunctiva following placement. These implants have a high tensile strength, yet they are malleable. This allows easy sculpting of the anterior surface of the implant. They may be used with or without a wrapping material.

Exposure of a porous implant necessitates immediate correction. Pegging was used in a trial to increase motility, however most oculoplastic surgeons no longer support implant pegging.

The choice of the implant, the implant size, its placement, gentle tissue handling, attention to creation of fornices with adequate conjunctival lining, proper upper and lower eyelid positioning and correction of any laxity are all important parts of the surgical planning and execution.

Though dermis fat graft is not considered often as a conventional orbital implant, it is an excellent material for implantation of pediatric anophthalmic sockets and fulfills most of the criteria of an ideal implant. Dermis fat graft is preferred in children with anophthalmic socket with both volume loss and conjunctival shortening (surface loss). It is also preferred in reconstruction of irradiated sockets where the vascularity is compromised and there is a higher

possibility of extrusion of alloplastic implant. However, fat atrophy can cause late volume loss in adults implanted with dermis fat graft.

Finally a custom–made prosthesis is fabricated. Most modern ocular protheses are made using polymethyl methacrylate (PMMA).

Orbital Implants and Prosthesis

1. Indications for enucleation, All are correct except:
   A. Intraocular malignancy
   B. Painful blind eye
   C. Severely traumatized eye
   D. Endophthalmitis.
2. The advantage of evisceration, one is false:
   A. Less disruption of orbital anatomy
   B. Less motility of prosthesis
   C. Better treatment of endophthalmitis
   D. Technically is a simple procedure.
3. Causes of contracted socket, one is false:
   A. Radiation treatment
   B. Extrusion of an enucleated implant
   C. Severe initial injury
   D. Removal of the conformer for short period.
4. The primary advantage of nonporous compared to porous orbital implant is:
   A. Better orbital volume replacement
   B. Lower exposure rates
   C. Increased implant stability
   D. Better prosthesis motility.
5. Enucleation in childhood, one is false:
   A. Associated with under development of the bony orbit
   B. Autogenous dermis fat graft have been shown to grow along with expanding orbit
   C. Using implants that exert maximal tension on tissues allow the orbital bone to grow
   D. Loss of volume of the orbit occurs when dermis fat graft is used as an implant in adults.
6. True statement regarding enucleation is:
   A. Indicated for primary intraocular tumor
   B. Cannot be performed under local anesthesia

C. Scleral shell trail can be an alternative to enculeation for non painful disfigured eyes

D. Early enucleation is indicated for all severely traumatized eyes.

7. The following is a complication of an anophthalmic socket:
   A. Excessive fibrosis leading to increase orbital volume
   B. Deep superior sulcus
   C. Eyelids fusion
   D. Excessive vascularization.

8. When an enucleation is performed in a child:
   A. The implant should not be placed until the child is 7 years old
   B. A dermis–fat graft should be avoided because it does not grow with the orbit
   C. The optic nerve should be cut flush at the posterior sclera when retinoblastoma is present
   D. An adult size implant should be placed as soon as possible to promote orbital growth.

9. The least likely indication for exenteration is:
   A. Intraocular malignant melanoma that extended outside the globe with evidence of distant metastasis
   B. Management of epithelial tumors of the lacrimal gland
   C. Destructive tumors extending from the sinus to the orbit
   D. Primary orbital malignancy that do not respond to non surgical treatment modalities.

10. Regarding exenteration, one is false:
    A. Considered in management of recurrent rhabdomyosarcoma non responding to radio and chemotherapy
    B. Total exenteration is the removal of all intraorbital soft tissues with or without the skin of the eye lids
    C. Fixation of osseo-integrated implant is achieved with glue
    D. The exenteration prosthesis usually do not blink or move.

11. Characters of orbital implants, one is false:
    A. Inert spherical implants usually provide comfort
    B. Hydroxyapatite and porous implants allow for drilling and placement of a peg
    C. Pegging is usually carried out one month after the enucleation
    D. Pegged porous implants have the higher rates of postoperative complications.

12. Enucleation is indicated in, one is false:
    A. Retinoblastoma
    B. Panophthalmitis
    C. Ciliary staphyloma
    D. Penetrating injury of the eye with no hope of vision.

13. Regarding exenteration, one is true:
    A. Considered in management of huge rhabdomyosarcoma
    B. Total exentration is the removal of all intraocular tissue with or without the skin of eyelids
    C. Fixating of ossoointegrated implant is achieved with screw
    D. The exenteration prosthesis usually blink and move.

14. Causes of contracted socket, one is false:
    A. Chemotherapy treatment
    B. Extrusion of an enucleated implant
    C. Poor surgical technique
    D. Multiple socket operations.

15. In cases of implant extrusion following enucleation or evisceration, which is false;
    A. Early extrusion is associated with poor wound closure
    B. Early extrusion is associated with implant that is too small
    C. Late extrusion is associated with tumor recurrences
    D. Late extrusion is associated with conjunctival cyst.

16. Evisceration is contraindicated in:
    A. Endophthalmitis
    B. Atrophia bulbi
    C. Massive vitreous seedling retinal tumors
    D. Absolute glaucoma.

17. Blind painful left eye has secondarily developed perforation of the cornea. The surgical procedure of choice is,
    A. Evisceratiom with Keratectomy
    B. Evisceration without keratectomy
    C. Enucleation
    D. Exentration.

18. The most common postoperative complication of enucleation is
    A. Socket contracture
    B. Enophthalmos
    C. Superior sulcus deformity
    D. Extrusion of implant.

19. Regarding Evisceration for blind painful eyes, which is incorrect:
    A. The procedure is appropriate even in the setting of endophthalmitis
    B. There is a low risk of developing granulomatous inflammation in the other eye
    C. Posterior incisions in the sclera allow for placing a larger orbital implant
    D. The cornea may be retained provided the epithelium is removed.

20. A patient undergoes an uncomplicated enucleation for a blind, painful eye. A hydroxyapatite implant is placed in the socket. Six weeks after surgery, the patient's examination shows a well-healed socket with a deep superior and inferior fornix. Movement of the orbital implant is excellent. However, the patient is disappointed that the prosthesis does not move well and asks if any improvements are possible. You discuss the option of pegging the implant, which can be coupled to the prosthesis and improve prosthesis movement. What is the most appropriate next step?
    A. Schedule the patient for the next available surgical date
    B. Order MRI with contrast of the orbit
    C. Order a bone scan of the orbit
    D. Schedule the patient for a return visit in 3 months.

21. Which of the following would not cause discharge in patients with an anophthalmic socket and ocular prosthesis?
    A. An old prosthesis
    B. Dry socket

C. Bacterial conjunctivitis
D. Eyelid malposition.

22. What is an advantage of evisceration over enucleation?
    A. Lower risk of sympathetic ophthalmia
    B. Better treatment of endophthalmitis
    C. No need for placement of orbital implant
    D. Better histopathologic examination of intraocular contents.

23. Which of the following is not a reported complication of hydroxyapatite implants?
    A. HIV transmission from the donor sclera
    B. Exposure of the hydroxyapatite surface
    C. Chronic bacterial infection in the implant
    D. Migration and extrusion of the implant.

24. A patient has an NLP and painful eye shortly after treatment for chronic endophthalmitis. When evaluating the surgical options, which technique is preferable?
    A. Enucleation
    B. Evisceration
    C. Subtotal exenteration
    D. Total exenteration.

25. Regarding hydroxyapatite orbital implant after enucleation, which is incorrect:
    A. Is usually wrapped in donor sclera
    B. Receives the four rectus muscles
    C. Requires a peg to produce maximal movement of the implant
    D. May be rejected by the body's immune system.

26. Regarding evisceration, which is incorrect:
    A. Is contraindicated in cases of suspected intraocular malignancy
    B. Always requires corneal removal
    C. Does not obviate the risk of sympathetic ophthalmia
    D. Is contraindicated if precise histopathologic examination of the globe is needed.

27. Complications of exenteration include all except:
    A. Severe blood loss
    B. "Phantom limb" pain from the cut optic nerve
    C. Skin graft infection
    D. Chronic sino-orbital fistulas.

28. Regarding pegging of an integrated implant, all are true except:
    A. Generally undergoes drilling 6 to 12 months after placement
    B. Improve prosthesis movement
    C. Markedly increase the incidence of complications
    D. Is the standard of care now.

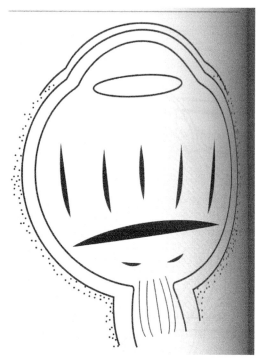

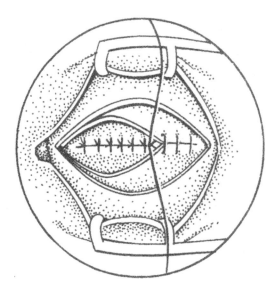

30. The above technique is used to allow:
    A. Suturing of the extra ocular muscles
    B. Fibrovascular ingrowth into a porous implant
    C. Insertion of a larger implant
    D. Drainage of any postoperative hemorrhage.

29. Regarding closure of evisceration, which is false:
    A. Must be done in multiple layers
    B. A running locking suture is used for the conjunctiva
    C. Sutures should be removed after 1 week
    D. Must eliminate potential space between the layers.

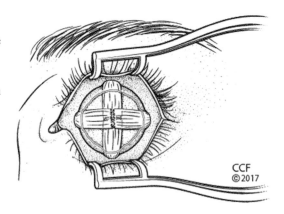

31. The above technique is:
    A. Primarily used in children
    B. Provides both volume and surface
    C. Allow for bony socket expansion
    D. Has a higher rate of infection.

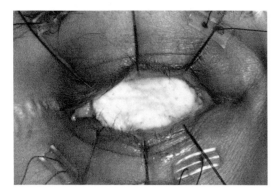

32. The above technique:
    A. The extraocular muscles can be sutured to it
    B. Grows with the growth of the child
    C. Has a higher exposure rate
    D. Can be used when vascularity is compromised.

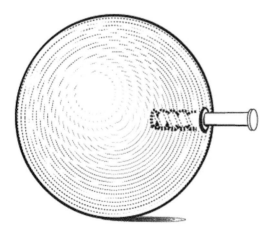

33. Regarding orbital implant size, which is false:
    A. Should provide at least 70% of the removed volume
    B. Is essentially determined preoperatively
    C. Is essentially determined intraoperatively
    D. Is smaller if wrapping is used.

34. Regarding orbital implant size, which is false:
    A. May require examining the other eye
    B. Depend on the surgical procedure used
    C. Takes the thickness of the prosthesis into consideration
    D. Is larger if the eye was staphylomatous.

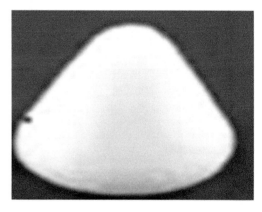

35. Implantation of the above implant design results in all except:
    A. Less risk of exposure
    B. More contact with orbital fat
    C. Easier surgical technique
    D. Insertion of a larger implant volume.

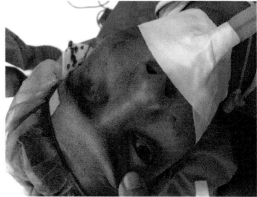

36. The above patient had a history of retino-blastoma treated by exenteration and radio-therapy, his best option now is:
    A. Insertion of a non integrated implant
    B. Insertion of an integrated implant
    C. Use of a dermis fat graft
    D. Use of a pedicled local flap.
37. During evisceration, removal of the uvea is made easier by:
    A. Keratectomy
    B. Disinsertion of the scleral spur
    C. Expansion sclerotomies
    D. Bipolar cautery.
38. During evisceration, the risk of sympathetic ophthalmia is further reduced by the use of:
    A. 70% alcohol
    B. Hydrogen peroxide
    C. Betadine
    D. Iodoform gauze.
39. The ideal size of the ocular prosthesis is:
    A. 2 mL
    B. 2.5 mL
    C. 3 mL
    D. 3.5 mL.

40. Which of the following is recommended for 6-monthly follow-up of patients who have had enucleation for ocular melanoma?
    A. CT abdomen
    B. PET CT
    C. Serological liver function tests
    D. Ultrasound of the liver.

Answers of Orbital Implants and Prosthesis

1	D	16	C	31	D
2	B	17	A	32	C
3	D	18	C	33	C
4	B	19	D	34	D
5	C	20	C	35	C
6	C	21	B	36	D
7	B	22	B	37	B
8	D	23	A	38	B
9	A	24	B	39	B
10	C	25	D	40	D
11	C	26	B		
12	B	27	B		
13	C	28	D		
14	A	29	C		
15	B	30	C		

Oculoplasty Interactions with Other Specialities

10

Essam A. El Toukhy

The interaction between oculoplasty and other ophthalmic subspecialities is more than with any other ophthalmic subspeciality. With pediatric ophthalmology; The development of the lids plays a crucial role for the normal function of the eyes as well as the impact of the cosmetic appearance on the functional and psychological welfare of the child. The whole spectrum of lid anomalies is an essential part of oculoplasty. Ptosis, lid colobomas and epiblepharon are just examples. Also, The position of the upper and lower lids is usually changed after any surgery on the extraocular muscles most likely due to the close embryological, anatomical and innervational relations between the lid muscles, extraocular muscles and orbital connective tissues. This directly reflects on the management of patients requiring strabismus surgery and lid surgery.

Corneal Refractive Surgery is intimately related to Oculoplasty as the cornea is an integral part of the ocular surface and is affected by the anatomical and functional status of the ocular adnexa and tear production and function. Preoperative evaluation of patients seeking refractive correction can guide the surgeon to the proper timing of surgery, select the best technique for each patient and allow him to treat any preexisting conditions that may lead to certain operative challenges or possible postoperative complications. Abnormalities in lid margin, palpebral fissure, blinking pattern or lid inflammations are such examples. Tear film evaluation both quantitatively and qualitatively is essential. Intraoperative challenges related to ocular adnexa should be anticipated, prevented and/or properly managed. Postoperative changes in corneal sensation and their effect on tear production, corneal healing and patient subjective symptoms of dry eye and finally on his quality of vision and satisfaction should be properly understood and managed. Failure to identify and manage these challenges before, during and after refractive surgery may lead to serious complications and can affect the final visual outcome and patient satisfaction.

Ptosis, whether primary or residual after lid surgery, has direct impact on patient refraction by pressing on the upper cornea leading to corneal astigmatism and abnormal topography. If it is severe enough to cover the pupil since birth, it may lead to amblyopia that cannot be corrected by refractive surgery. Ptosis or tight lids, if missed or left untreated, may also affect the Lasik flap postoperatively leading to flap wrinkles or striae. Lagophthalmos can follow facial palsy or be a sequel of lid surgery like ptosis, entropion or lid tumors. It may result in unstable tear film, exposure keratitis, dry eye or even corneal opacity. Lid margin abnormalities like

E. A. El Toukhy (✉)
Oculoplasty Service, Cairo University, Cairo, Egypt
e-mail: eeltoukhy@yahoo.com

© The Author(s), under exclusive license to Springer Nature Switzerland AG 2021
E. A. El Toukhy (ed.), *Oculoplasty for Ophthalmologists*, https://doi.org/10.1007/978-3-030-68469-3_10

143

rubbing lashes, entropion or ectropion should be checked as they may lead to intraoperative difficulties of proper corneal exposure or pressing against the LASIK flap distorting it.

Lid margin inflammation like blepharitis and Meibomian gland dysfunction (MGD) should not be missed during preoperative examination. They can affect the accuracy and reliability of preoperative investigations like corneal topography and tomography leading to wrong decision making. They may also lead to serious intraoperative challenges by pouring meibomian secretions on the corneal surface or under the lasik flap. These secretions may interfere with femtolaser pathway and gas bubble formation, block excimer laser ablation or become trapped under a Lasik flap or in a SMILE pocket. In rare cases, they may also lead to diffuse lamellar keratitis (DLK) or interface debris. All types of blepharitis can also be a source of postoperative inflammation like diffuse lamellar keratitis (DLK).

Patients with floppy eyelids and sleep apnea are also more liable to eye rubbing with its serious effect on Lasik flap leading to flap wrinkles, flap striae or even flap displacement. Both infrequent blinking and excessive blinking can affect the ocular surface health, tear stability and tear clearance. Not only can this exaggerate symptoms of dry eye but can also affect postoperative healing and flap adherence, especially in surface ablation procedures. Blinking abnormalities are very common in patients who have been contact lens wearers for a long time with subsequent diminished corneal sensation and lack of the stimulus to blink.

Above all, the most important preoperative examination is for ocular surface health, tear volume, tear stability and tear clearance as indicators of dry eye disease (DED). Tear film abnormalities whether epiphora or unstable tear film seriously affect preoperative investigations including placido-based corneal topography, optical scheimflug tomography or all types of wavefront aberrometry measuring systems. This can lead to a false diagnosis of irregular corneal surface like keratoconus or can mask an existing abnormality. It is now advised to have a dry eye clinic in each refractive surgery center to ensure proper diagnosis and management of dry eye patients or those at a higher risk of developing it and treating them before they undergo refractive surgery.

In patients with persistent lid problems like lagophthalmos, infrequent blinking or lid margin abnormalities, it is better to avoid Lasik and shift to either surface ablation, refractive lenticule extraction (SMILE) or to intra-ocular surgery like phakic IOLs. Those cases can also benefit from intra-operative punctal occlusion by temporary punctal plugs to keep normal tears.

Glaucoma, as a disease entity, can affect the cosmetic aspect of the eye in multiple ways. The disease in itself can be associated with angry red looking eyes, due to either high eye pressure or as a side effect of glaucoma medications. In advanced cases the disease itself or as a result of complicated surgery can result in a shrunken phthisic eye, or an enlarged staphylomatous one.

Effects of preservatives have been indicated as a causative factor of ocular surface disease (OSD) associated with ophthalmic antiglaucomatous agent administration. More than 60% of patients with glaucoma have signs and symptoms of OSD.

Conjunctival allergy, conjunctival hyperemia, corneal epithelial disorders, and blepharitis are common adverse reactions associated with most anti glaucoma eyedrops. With prostaglandin analogs, patients may also have eyelash bristling/lengthening, vellus hair, eyelid pigmentation, iris pigmentation, and deepening of the upper eyelid sulcus (DUES).

Ocular adverse reactions associated with carbonic anhydrase inhibitors include conjunctival allergy, conjunctival hyperemia, corneal epithelial disorders, blepharitis, Stevens–Johnson syndrome, and toxic epidermal necrosis. With Rho khinase inhibitors, The most frequent adverse events were ocular: conjunctival hyperemia, conjunctival hemorrhage, and cornea verticillata.

Finally, glaucoma surgeries can result in ptosis or upper eyelid retraction due to mechanical or myogenic mechanisms.

A variety of conditions may present with symptoms and signs that overlap between the subspecialties of oculoplastics and neuro-ophthalmology.

Neuro-ophthalmic disorders affecting lid and ocular muscles as Myasthenia gravis or CPEO is a classic example of the interaction between oculoplasty and neuro ophthalmology. These disorders present commonly with ptosis and are usually first seen by the oculoplastic surgeon. The diagnosis of such conditions is based on the clinical presentations, serological and pharmacological tests and electrophysiological assessments Proper diagnosis and management requires co-management between both specialities.

Giant cell arteritis (GCA), also known as temporal arteritis, is one of the most important emergencies in ophthalmology because of its irreversible and devastating effect on vision in approximately half of patients. Temporal artery biopsy performed by an oculoplastic surgeon is the gold-standard for diagnosis and should be done in every patient where clinical suspicion is high; regardless of the results of any other test.

Horner syndrome (HS), an oculo-sympathetic palsy which includes the triad of eyelid ptosis, ipsilateral miosis and facial anhidrosis, is another example where the oculoplastic surgeon is involved in the diagnosis, localization and surgical management.

For idiopathic intracranial hypertension (IIH), Treatment and management requires multi-specialty team work. Optic nerve sheath fenestration (ONSF) surgery is usually performed by the oculoplastic surgeon on request by the neuro ophthalmologist.

Carotid cavernous sinus fistula (CCF), particularly the spontaneous type, should be considered in the differential diagnosis of Graves' ophthalmopathy, orbital cellulitis and idiopathic intra-orbital inflammation

The orbit is closely related anatomically to the paranasal sinuses. It is related superiorly to the frontal sinus, medially to the ethmoid sinuses, inferiorly to the maxillary sinus and posteromedially to the anterolateral wall of the sphenoid sinus. Owing to this close anatomic proximity, both can share same diseases, and/or extension from one of them to the other can occur.

A variety of diseases are unique in their ability to involve both the sinonasal (SN) cavities and the orbits. It is more common for SN pathology to affect the orbit than the reverse, and primary sinus pathology may initially present with predominantly orbital, rather than sinus, symptomatology.

Generally, there is more than one ocular symptom found in each patient with sinonasal disease extending to the orbit. Proptosis is the commonest occurring in about 60% of cases. The direction of proptosis is an important clue of the location of the involved sinus. Frontal sinus proptosis occurs inferiorly and is accompanied by swelling of the brow area. Direct lateral proptosis occurs in ethmoid sinus disease. With maxillary sinus pathology, the proptosis is upwards.

Other less common symptoms include ophthalmoplegia and visual loss. A decrease in visual acuity indicates of optic nerve involvement. The underlying pathophysiology may be caused by direct compression of the nerve fibers, non-perfusion of its blood vessels or inflammation/infection in proximity to the nerve.

Ophthalmoplegia can be caused by a mechanical restriction on extraocular muscles or nerves paresis. Force duction test can distinguish between both. Positive test denotes mechanical restrictions. Abnormal ocular motility can cause diplopia both at the primary gaze position and the position of the extremes gaze.

Disease entities affecting the sino-orbital region may arise primarily in the SN cavities, the orbits, or the surrounding bones; or they may result from secondary involvement by systemic disorders. Generally, sino-orbital pathologies can be classified broadly into four groups: (1) Infectious and inflammatory conditions; bacterial sinusitis and orbital cellulitis, fungal infections, mucoceles and the silent sinus syndrome (2) Granulomatous disease; GPA, sarcoidosis, and Rhinoscleroma (3) Fibro-osseous lesions; osteomas and fibrous dysplasia and (4) Neoplasms: particularly malignant sinus tumors.

Maxillofacial lesions involving the periorbital area include primarily trauma and oncological lesions. A thorough knowledge of bony landmarks, lymphatic drainage and routes of perineural invasion is a must for the oculoplastic surgeon.

Dermatological disorders can be reflected in the eye and the periorbital area. Various skin diseases can affect the skin of the periorbital area e.g. dermatitis, vitiligo, xanthelasma, hidrocystomas, syringomas, milia, etc. Other cutaneous disorders may have associated ocular involvement e.g. rosacea, port-wine stain and nevus of Ota. Some infectious diseases can affect both the skin and eyes e.g. herpes simplex and herpes zoster. Systemic diseases can have ocular, as well as, dermatological involvement e.g. amyloidosis, dermatomyositis, sarcoidosis and Bechet's disease. Periorbital dermatological procedures e.g. periorbital chemical peeling and laser procedures, and their expected complications, can be of interest to the oculoplastic surgeon.

The skin of the eyelid has a similar structure to the skin elsewhere in the body with some unique features. The eyelid skin is the thinnest in the body particularly the medial aspect of the upper eyelid. Glands in the eyelids include the sebaceous glands (meibomian glands and sebaceous gland of Zeis), and both eccrine and apocrine sweat glands (apocrine sweat gland of Moll). Terminal hair is also present in the form of eyebrow and eyelashes. Therefore, a wide variety of skin conditions that originate from these skin structures can present in the periorbital area. Periorbital skin diseases can be classified into melanocytic and vascular nevi, neoplastic, infectious, manifestations of systemic diseases, nevi and disorders of pigmentation and disorders of eyebrow and eyelashes.

Obtaining an incisional or excisional biopsy is a day to day procedure in oculoplasty. proper handling of the samples, preservation techniques and a presumed working diagnosis are essential. Eyelid lesions including melanocytic lesions and lymphoproliferative orbital lesions are amongst the common oculoplastic specimens requiring pathological differentiation. Immunohistochemistry and tumor markers diagnosis require special specimen handling.

Interaction with Other Specialities:

1. Recession of the inferior rectus results in:
   A. Narrowing of the palpebral fissure
   B. Widening of the palpebral fissure
   C. No effect on the palpebral fissure
   D. The effect will depend on the laxity of the canthal tendons.
2. Recession of the superior rectus results in:
   A. Narrowing of the palpebral fissure
   B. Widening of the palpebral fissure
   C. No effect on the palpebral fissure
   D. The effect will depend on the laxity of the canthal tendons.
3. Recession of the medial or lateral rectus results in:
   A. Narrowing of the palpebral fissure
   B. Widening of the palpebral fissure
   C. No effect on the palpebral fissure
   D. The effect will depend on the laxity of the canthal tendons.
4. Weakening procedures of the inferior oblique muscle results in:
   A. Narrowing of the palpebral fissure in upgaze
   B. Narrowing of the palpebral fissure in downgaze
   C. Widening of the palpebral fissure in upgaze
   D. Widening of the palpebral fissure in downgaze.
5. Ocular complications of craniosynostosis include all except:
   A. Exposure keratopathy
   B. Stabismus
   C. Proptosis
   D. Ptosis.
6. Craniosynostosis:
   A. Is usually syndromic
   B. Is mostly hereditary
   C. Usually presents at birth
   D. Usually requires simple observation in most cases.
7. Blepharophimosis, all are true except:
   A. Is mostly hereditary
   B. Usually presents at birth
   C. Usually requires simple observation in most cases
   D. Is usually syndromic.

8. Blepharophimosis can be associated with:
   A. Diabetes insipidus
   B. Early testicular failure
   C. Early ovarian failure
   D. Cardiac anomalies.

9. In craniosynostosis, the most serious manifestation is;
   A. Exposure keratopathy
   B. Proptosis
   C. Strabismus
   D. Raised intracranial pressure.

10. Goldenhar syndrome:
   A. Is due to an abnormality of chromosome 21
   B. Is due to maldevelopment of all branchial arches
   C. Is mainly ocular
   D. Epibulbar dermoids result in amblyopia.

11. All of the following are syndromes involving craniofacial synostosis *except*:
   A. Crouzon syndrome
   B. Treacher-Collins syndrome
   C. Apert syndrome
   D. Pfeiffer syndrome.

12. All of the following clinical findings can be associated with Goldenhar syndrome *except*:
   A. Eyelid colobomas
   B. Lipodermoids
   C. Duane syndrome
   D. Proptosis.

13. Which systemic condition is incorrectly paired with a skin lesion?
   A. Sturge-Weber syndrome (encephalotrigeminal angiomatosis)-nevus flammeus (port-wine stain)
   B. Ataxia-telangiectasia-cafe-au-lait spots
   C. Incontinentia pigmenti-hyperpigmented macules ("splashed paint")
   D. Tuberous sclerosis-facial angiofibromas (adenoma sebaceum).

14. Ptosis can affect a refractive procedure by causing all except:
   A. Tear film disturbance
   B. Abnormal topography
   C. Amblyopia
   D. Flap abnormalities.

15. MGD can affect a refractive procedure by causing all except;
   A. Tear film disturbance
   B. Exposure keratopathy
   C. Block laser pathway
   D. Entrapment under the flap.

16. MGD can result in all of the following complications following LASIK except:
   A. Delayed epithelialization
   B. DLK
   C. Infections
   D. Regression.

17. Which procedure produces most affection of corneal sensation:
   A. PRK
   B. PTK
   C. Lasik
   D. SMILE.

18. Risk factors for post LASIK dry eyes include all except:
   A. Prior use of contact lenses
   B. Thicker flap
   C. Deeper ablation
   D. Smaller error of refraction.

19. The silent sinus syndrome produces:
   A. Exophthalmos
   B. Enophthalmos
   C. Lid retraction
   D. Emphysema.

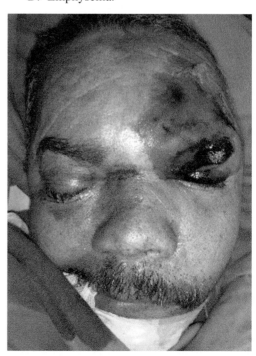

20. Regarding the above patient, all are true except:
    A. Patient idiabetic or immunocompromised
    B. It is fungal in origin
    C. Spreads rapidly with tissue necrosis
    D. Has an excellent prognosis.
21. In the above patient, all are true except
    A. Infection starts in the nose then spreads
    B. Spread to the orbit is late
    C. Palatal necrosis and perforation is common
    D. Intracranial spread can occur.

22. In the above patient, all are true except;
    A. The pathology is essentially vascular occlusion
    B. MRI can demonstrate fungal hyphae
    C. Early debridement is required
    D. IV antibiotics should be used immediately.

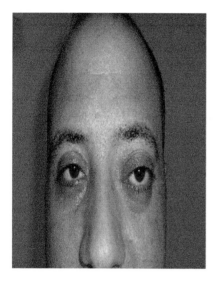
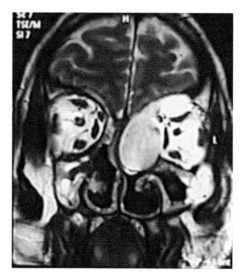

23. The above lesion:
    A. Originates from the sphenoid sinus
    B. Originates from the frontal and ethmoidal sinuses
    C. Originates from the lacrimal sac
    D. Originates from the nasal cavity.

24. All are true regarding the above lesion except:
    A. Benign in nature
    B. Malignant
    C. Progressive
    D. Must be removed asap.

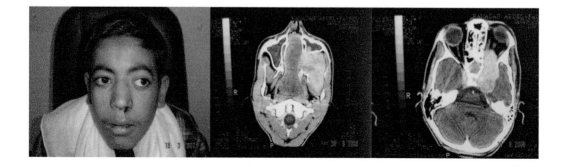

25. All are true about the above lesion except:
    A. It produces frog face deformity
    B. It arises from the nose and sinuses
    C. It is malignant
    D. It is more common in adolescent males.
26. The above lesion:
    A. Is highly vascular
    B. Extends through the inferior orbital fissure
    C. May require embolization before excision
    D. Has a poor prognosis.
27. Myasthenia gravis is due to:
    A. Presynaptic antibodies against acetylcholine
    B. Postsynaptic antibodies against acetylcholine
    C. Presynaptic antibodies against acetylcholine receptors
    D. Postsynaptic antibodies against acetylcholine receptors.
28. In myasthenia gravis; the following are normal except:
    A. Sensory functions
    B. Pupillary reactions
    C. Accommodation
    D. Recti muscles.
29. All the following tests can be used to diagnose myasthenia except:
    A. Sleep test
    B. Dark test
    C. Ice test
    D. Fatigue test.
30. All the following tests can be used to diagnose myasthenia except:
    A. Tensilon test
    B. Edrophonium test
    C. Atropine test
    D. EMG testing
31. Investigations to diagnose myasthenia include all except:
    A. Serum AChr antibodies
    B. EMG
    C. Nystagmography
    D. Single fiber EMG.
32. Mestinon (pyridostigmine) is:
    A. Acetylcholine agonist
    B. Acetylcholine inhibtor

C. Acetylcholine esterase agonist
D. Acetylcholine esterase inhibitor.
33. Giant cell arteritis involves:
    A. Small-sized arteries
    B. Mid and large-sized arteries
    C. All types of arteries
    D. All types of vessels.
34. The most common symptom in giant cell arteritis is:
    A. Jaw claudication
    B. Headache
    C. Visual loss
    D. Cranial nerve palsy.
35. The most specific symptom in giant cell arteritis is:
    A. Jaw claudication
    B. Headache
    C. Visual loss
    D. Cranial nerve palsy.
36. Combined sensitivity of ESR and CRP in giant cell arteritis is:
    A. 70%
    B. 80%
    C. 90%
    D. 99%.
37. The gold standard test for giant cell arteritis is;
    A. Combined ESR and CRP
    B. Carotid angiography
    C. Temporal artery biopsy
    D. Fluorescein angiography.
38. Horner syndrome includes all except:
    A. Ptosis
    B. Proptosis
    C. Miosis
    D. Anhydrosis.
39. First order neuron Horner syndrome is mostly:
    A. Traumatic
    B. Vascular
    C. Tumor related
    D. Postoperative.
40. Second order neuron Horner syndrome can be due to all except:
    A. Traumatic
    B. Vascular
    C. Tumor related
    D. Congenital.

41. Third order neuron Horner syndrome can be due to all except:
    A. Traumatic
    B. Vascular
    C. Tumor related
    D. Congenital.

42. The pupil in Horner syndrome exhibits all except:
    A. Miosis
    B. Dilation lag
    C. Poor response to Apraconidine
    D. Poor response to cocaine.

43. Intracranial pressure of above—is needed to diagnose idiopathic intracranial hypertension:
    A. 15 mm water
    B. 20 mm water
    C. 25 mm water
    D. 30 mm water.

44. Use of all of the following drugs can lead to increased intracranial pressure except:
    A. Tetracycline
    B. Vitamin D
    C. Vitamin A
    D. Isotretinoin.

45. Indications for surgery in Idiopathic intracranial hypertension include all except:
    A. Male gender
    B. Bilateral affection
    C. Progressive field loss
    D. Central visual loss.

46. Systemic examination of a patient with chronic progressive external ophthalmoplegia is necessary to exclude:
    A. Hepatic disease
    B. Neurological disease
    C. Cardiac disease
    D. Renal disease.

47. Perineural spread is more common to occur with:
    A. Basal cell carcinoma
    B. Squamous cell carcinoma
    C. Sebaceous cell carcinoma
    D. Malignant melanoma.

48. Topical medications for glaucoma can result in ocular surface disease in about:
    A. 40% of patients
    B. 50% of patients

C. 60% of patients
D. 70% of patients.

49. Oculoplastic side effects of prostaglandin analogs include all except:
    A. Deepening of the superior sulcus
    B. Eyelid pigmentation
    C. Eyelid retraction
    D. Eyelash lengthening.

50. Oculoplastic side effects of ROCK inhibitors include:
    A. Conjunctival hemorrhage
    B. Eyelid pigmentation
    C. Blepharitis
    D. Eyelash lengthening.

51. Oculoplastic complications of glaucoma surgery can include all except:
    A. Ptosis
    B. Lid retraction
    C. Ectropion
    D. Dry eyes.

52. What is the least likely ocular complication from endoscopic sinus surgery?
    A. Diplopia
    B. Blindness
    C. Tearing
    D. Ptosis.

53. What is the most common eyelid condition associated with the use of topical latanoprost?
    A. Depigmentation of the iris and periocular skin
    B. Eyelid margin necrosis
    C. Hyperpigmentation of periocular skin and eyelid-margin hyperemia
    D. Severe hirsutism of periocular skin.

54. Which nutritional supplement should be avoided prior to eyelid and orbital surgery because of its effect on platelets?
    A. Eicosapentaenoic acid (fish oil)
    B. Echinacea
    C. Glucosamine
    D. Valerian.

55. Which sinus system aerates first?
    A. Maxillary
    B. Frontal
    C. Sphenoid
    D. Ethmoid.

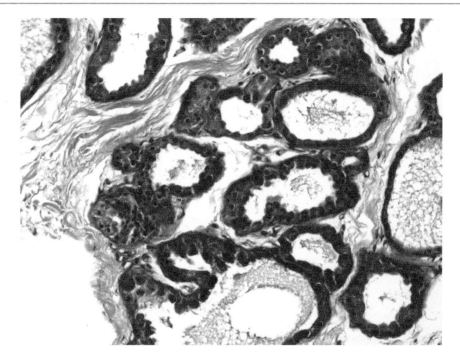

56. The above lesion is;
    A. Chalazion
    B. Hidrocystoma
    C. Keratoacanthoma
    D. Hemangioma.

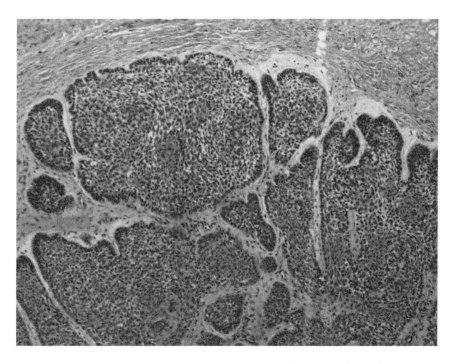

57. The above lesion is:
    A. Basal cell carcinoma
    B. Squamous cell carcinoma
    C. Sebaceous cell carcinoma
    D. Malignant melanoma.

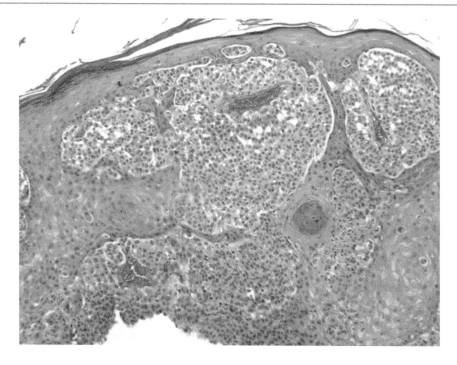

58. The above lesion is:
    A. Basal cell carcinoma
    B. Squamous cell carcinoma
    C. Sebaceous cell carcinoma
    D. Malignant melanoma.

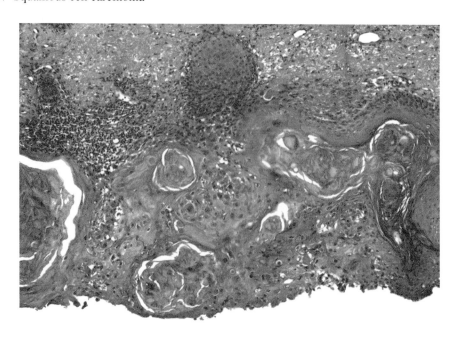

59. The above lesion is:
    A. Basal cell carcinoma
    B. Squamous cell carcinoma
    C. Sebaceous cell carcinoma
    D. Malignant melanoma.

60. Satellite lesions occur in:
    A. Basal cell carcinoma
    B. Squamous cell carcinoma
    C. Sebaceous cell carcinoma
    D. Malignant melanoma.

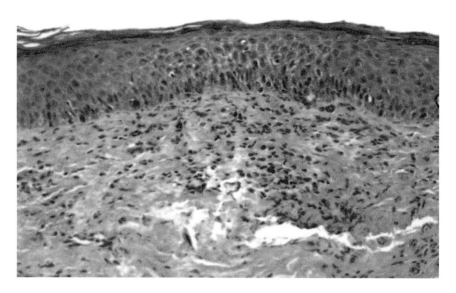

61. The above lesion is:
    A. Pigmented basal cell carcinoma
    B. Lentigo maligna
    C. Intradermal nevus
    D. Malignant melanoma.

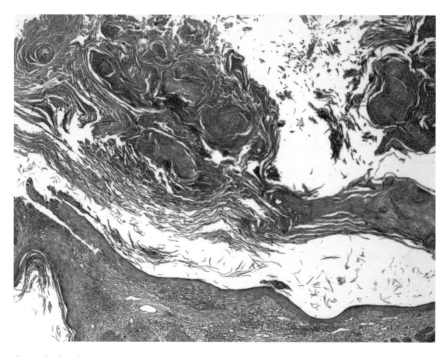

62. The above lesion is;
    A. Chalazion
    B. Hidrocystoma
    C. Keratoacanthoma
    D. Hemangioma.

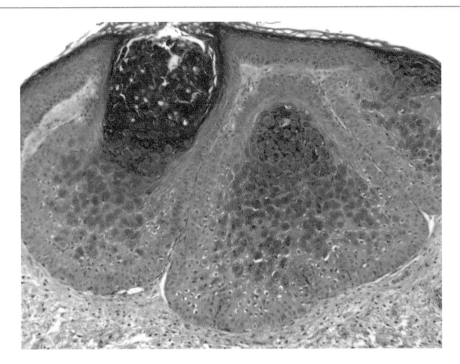

63. The above lesion is;
    A. Chalazion
    B. Xanthelasma
    C. Schwannoma
    D. Molluscum contagiosum.

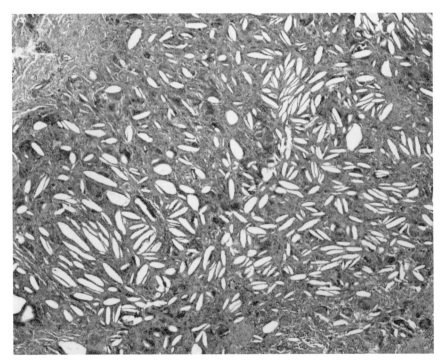

64. The above lesion is;
    A. Chalazion
    B. Xanthelasma
    C. Schwannoma
    D. Hemangioma.

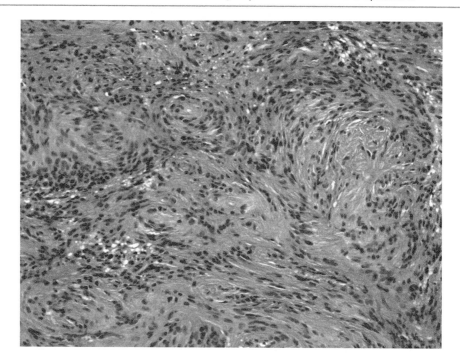

65. The above lesion is:
    A. Chalazion
    B. Xanthelasma
    C. Schwannoma
    D. Hemangioma.

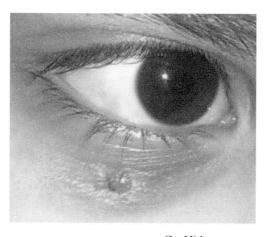

66. The above lesion is:
    A. Herpes simplex
    B. Molluscum contagiosum
    C. Hidrocystoma
    D. Syringoma.

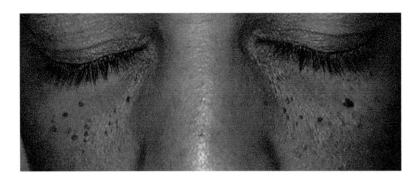

67. The above lesion is:
    A. Milia
    B. Rosacea

    C. Multiple skin tags
    D. Dermatosis papulosa nigra.

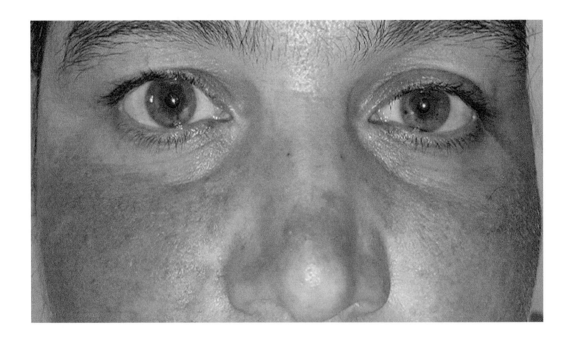

68. The above lesion is:
    A. Port wine stain
    B. Rosacea

    C. Contact dermatitis
    D. Atopic dermatitis.

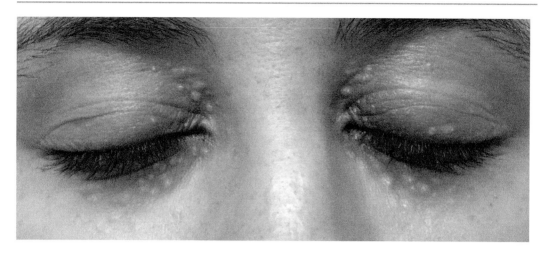

69. The above lesion is:
    A. Herpes simplex
    B. Syringomas
    C. Multiple skin tags
    D. Multiple hidrocystomas.

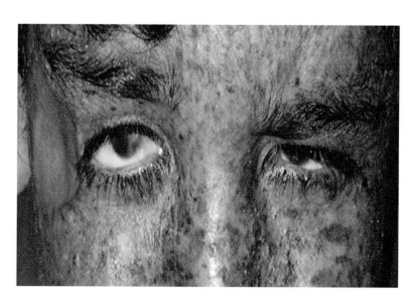

70. The above lesion is:
    A. Tuberous sclerosis
    B. Xeroderma pigmentosa
    C. Icthyosis
    D. Dermatosis papulosa nigra.
71. Eyelid halos (periorbital hyperpigmenta-
    tion), may be due to all except:
    A. The shadowing effect
    B. Tear trough depression
    C. Genetic susceptibility
    D. Lack of sleep.

72. Management of eyelid halos include all
    except:
    A. Peeling
    B. Fillers
    C. Blepharoplasty
    D. Botox.
73. All the following injections can be used to
    treat eyelid halos except:
    A. Fillers
    B. Botox
    C. Platelets–rich plasma
    D. Vitamin C.

74. According to the direction; Epicanthus can be all except:
    A. Tarsalis
    B. Lateralis
    C. Inversus
    D. Palpebralis.
75. The CSF in pseudotumor cerebri can show:
    A. High protein
    B. High cells
    C. High ph
    D. High pressure.
76. The surgical procedure of choice in CPEO is:
    A. Levator resection
    B. Muller resection
    C. Frontalis sling
    D. Frontalis flap.
77. The frontalis sling material used in CPEO must be:
    A. Synthetic
    B. Autologus
    C. Easily removed
    D. Permanent.
78. A characteristic radiological feature in carotid cavernous fistula is:
    A. Extraocular muscle enlargement
    B. Superior ophthalmic vein enlargement
    C. Orbital fat hypertrophy
    D. Internal carotid artery aneurysm.

79. The preservative commonly associated with OSD is:
    A. Polyquaternium
    B. Polyvinyl alcohol
    C. Benzalkonium chloride
    D. Sodium Purite.

Answers of Oculoplasty Interactions with Other Specialities

1	B	21	B	41	D	61	B
2	B	22	D	42	C	62	C
3	B	23	B	43	C	63	D
4	A	24	B	44	B	64	B
5	D	25	C	45	B	65	C
6	C	26	D	46	C	66	B
7	D	27	D	47	B	67	D
8	C	28	D	48	C	68	B
9	D	29	B	49	C	69	B
10	D	30	C	50	A	70	B
11	B	31	C	51	C	71	D
12	D	32	D	52	D	72	D
13	B	33	B	53	C	73	B
14	A	34	B	54	A	74	B
15	B	35	A	55	A	75	D
16	D	36	D	56	B	76	C
17	C	37	C	57	A	77	C
18	D	38	B	58	D	78	B
19	B	39	B	59	B	79	C
20	D	40	D	60	C		

Thyroid Eye Disease

Thyroid Eye Disease

Essam A. El Toukhy

Thyroid eye disease (TED) is an autoimmune condition with an active and inactive phase resulting in proptosis, eyelid retraction, and periorbital edema of varying severity. Symptoms range from mild eye irritation to vision loss from compressive optic neuropathy requiring medical and possibly acute surgical intervention. Active disease typically lasts one to three years before burn-out occurs; reactivation and irreversible vision loss is uncommon. An ophthalmologist can be of unique benefit to the patient in three valuable ways: (1) early diagnosis and referral for systemic treatment, (2) protection against the vision threatening effects of the disease, and (3) restoration of the patient's natural appearance.

TED is the most common cause of unilateral and bilateral proptosis. Women are six times more likely than men to have TED, and smoking is strongly associated with severity and risk of disease. Age has a first peak early in the third to fourth decade of life and a second peak in the mid-60s. The course usually follows the typical one described by Rundle: early progression, peak of inflammation at 6–24 months, followed by an inactive phase. Only 5–10% of patients have reactivation. Patients have eye irritation, edema, and finally proptosis from thickening of the extraocular muscles or orbital fat. The majority of patients with TED will experience mild disease with the most common presentation being erythema and eyelid retraction. The systemic effects of the disease should be managed with the patient's primary care doctor or an endocrinologist.

Pathologically, the key cell involved is the orbital fibroblast, which has a CD40 marker. This marker allows T cells to bind and upregulate the fibroblast's production of certain inflammatory markers (IL-6, IL-8, and prostaglandin E2). This upregulation results in deposition of hyaluronan and glycosaminoglycans (GAGs) to be deposited throughout the orbit and in the muscles. While this explains the thickening of the muscles, the orbital fat enlarges by a different mechanism. These various markers are the targets of several treatment modalities, one of which is teprotumumab.

It should be noted that TED is an autoimmune disease, not an endocrinal one. Testing only for thyroid hormones is non-conclusive and can be misleading. Testing for antibodies is more useful and is mandatory.

The clinical activity score (CAS) is a series of symptoms including pain in the orbit, pain with eye movements, redness of eyelids or conjunctiva, impaired movement or vision, and swelling of the eyelids, conjunctiva, caruncle or orbit (increasing proptosis). Each is given a point that when added together correlates with responsiveness to corticosteroids: the higher the

E. A. El Toukhy (✉)
Oculoplasty Service, Cairo University, Cairo, Egypt
e-mail: eeltoukhy@yahoo.com

© The Author(s), under exclusive license to Springer Nature Switzerland AG 2021
E. A. El Toukhy (ed.), *Oculoplasty for Ophthalmologists*, https://doi.org/10.1007/978-3-030-68469-3_11

159

score, the more likely symptoms will improve with medications.

All patients with TED benefit from maintenance in a euthyroid state. Coordinated care with an endocrinologist should be maintained throughout the patient's course. Concomitant steroids should be administered to all patients with TED that undergo radioactive iodine ablation (RAI). Similarly, patients with active disease, both moderate to severe disease and sight-threatening disease can be treated with oral or IV corticosteroids. Typically, a high dose of 1mg/kg until resolution followed by slow taper.

To avoid systemic steroids, or if the inflammatory process does not resolve or returns when the oral corticosteroids are finished, intraorbital intermediate acting steroids (Triamcinalone) or long-acting steroids (Dexamethasone) have been used successfully as an alternative to the systemic steroids for reduced morbidity.

Most recently, teprotumumab is a human insulin-like growth factor I (IGF-I) receptor inhibitory monoclonal antibody. Patients who were treated had significant reduction in proptosis and CAS score as well as improvement in quality of life at 6 months and a response as soon as 6 weeks without clinically significant side effects.

Vision loss or threatened vision loss is treated with decompression surgery. Up to three walls may be decompressed: the lateral wall, the floor, and the medial wall.

If patients have diplopia after reaching the chronic phase or after decompression, this should be repaired prior to eyelid surgery. Inferior rectus recession can create or exacerbate lower eyelid retraction. Lid restorative surgery to reconstruct their natural look should be undertaken afterwards. Common surgeries include recession of the upper and lower eyelids, mostly transconjunctivally. Blepharoplasty can benefit the patient both in terms of dermatochalasis improvement and to facilitate dissection superiorly via a lid crease incision to debulk some of the enlarged or thickened eyebrow fat pad inferior to the eyebrow cilia. The lower eyelid retraction can be repaired with or without a spacer to elevate the eyelid.

Thyroid Eye Diseases

1. Regarding clinical features of thyroid eye disease, one is false:
   A. Lid retraction is the most common sign
   B. More likely asymmetric
   C. More common in females
   D. Severity of the disease parallel serum level of T4 or T3.

2. Poor prognosis for orbitopathy in thyroid eye disease is associated with, one is false:
   A. Old male patient
   B. Perorbital myxedema
   C. Acropachy
   D. Myasthenia gravis.

3. Regarding treatment options for lid retraction in thyroid eye disease, one is false:
   A. Mild lid retraction often resolve spontaneously
   B. Six months of disease stability should be passed before surgical intervention is indicated
   C. Lid splitting, lateral tarsorrhaphy with recession of lid retractors is indicated if the patient have lateral flare
   D. Spacer graft is of no value in treatment of lower lid retraction.

4. Regarding orbital decompression in thyroid ophthalmopathy the most appropriate statement is:
   A. It is indicated when radiological evidence of swollen extraocular muscles is present
   B. It allows the swollen extraocular muscles to expand into periorbital space
   C. Orbital floor decompression can exacerbate lagophthalmos
   D. Removal of orbital fat during decompression exacerbate lid ptosis.

5. In the surgical treatment of upper lid retraction due to thyroid associated ophthalmopathy, one of the following statements is correct:
   A. Contraindicated in exposure keratopathy
   B. Evidence of disease stability must be documented prior to surgery in the presence of exposure keratopathy
   C. Can be corrected with excision of Müller muscle
   D. Lateral tarsorrhapy is the surgical modality of choice.

6. In a patient with Grave's ophthalmopathy and strabismus, how long should the angle of deviation be stable before performing the surgical correction?
   A. 1 month
   B. 3 months
   C. 6 months
   D. 1 year.

7. A patient who is a known case of Diabetes type 1 and hypertension presents with history of decreased vision with abnormal visual field, and RAPD in OD. His blood work up shows marked hyperthyroid status, high blood sugar level of 15 mmol/L and normal renal function. General anaesthesia is felt to be risky as the patient is on the brink of a thyroid storm. What would be the most appropriate management modality for vision-threatening thyroid ophthalmopathy in this case?
   A. Intravenous corticosteroid
   B. Lateral tarsorrhaphy
   C. Orbital radiation
   D. Oral corticosteroid.

8. Regarding orbital decompression in thyroid eye disease, one is false:
   A. Indicated to restore globe position even if there is no sight threatening conditions
   B. Indicated if radiotherapy was not effective
   C. Fat versus bone decompression is based on patient's age
   D. Orbital surgery should precede strabismus surgery.

9. During decompression of the orbital floor, diplopia and dystopia can be minimized by preserving:
   A. The palatine bone
   B. The bone between the medial wall and the floor
   C. The zygomatic bone
   D. The ethmoidal bone.

10. The correct order of surgical procedures in thyroid-associated orbitopathy is:
    A. Orbital wall decompression, then eyelid surgery, then strabismus surgery
    B. Orbital wall decompression, then strabismus surgery, then eyelid surgery

    C. Strabismus surgery, then eyelid surgery, then orbital wall decompression
    D. Eyelid surgery, then orbital wall decompression, then strabismus surgery.

11. In thyroid eye disease:
    A. The medial and inferior recti are the most commonly affected extraocular muscles
    B. Optic nerve fenestration is useful in patients with optic nerve compression
    C. Downgaze is most commonly affected in patients with ocular motility problems
    D. The thyroid function test always shows hyperthyroidism.

12. A patient with congestive thyroid orbitopathy had been taking 60 mg daily oral prednisone for 9 months. The dosage was tapered to 0 mg over a week. The patient now reports nausea, vomiting, muscle aches and pain. Initial considerations include which of the following?
    A. Acute adrenal insufficiency
    B. Thyroid storm
    C. Acute thyroid insufficiency
    D. Steroid induced diabetes.

13. Regarding thyroid eye disease, the incorrect statement is;
    A. 20% of patients with thyroid eye disease will need surgical treatment
    B. Radiation therapy should be avoided in patients with diabetes
    C. Orbital decompression should be done after strabismus surgery
    D. Smokers appear to be at greater risk for exacerbation of eye disease after radioactive iodine therapy.

14. The most common cause of unilateral proptosis in adults is;
    A. Lymphoma
    B. Cavernous hemangioma
    C. Thyroid eye disease
    D. Meningioma.

15. A 56 years old female with Grave's ophthalmopathy, on orbital CT most likely to be found is;
    A. An increased amount of orbital fat in the presence of normal size extra ocular muscles

B. Diffuse fusiform enlargement of extra ocular muscle belly and tendon.

C. Pressure erosion of lateral orbital rim from enlarged muscles

D. Chronic ethmoidal and maxillary sinusitis.

16. Orbital decompression in case of dysthyroid ophthalmopathy is indicated in the following except;
   A. Severe proptosis
   B. Optic neuropathy
   C. Early active phase
   D. Glucocorticoid side effects.

17. Features of thyroid ophthalmopathy include all except:
   A. External ophthalmoplegia
   B. Internal ophthalmoplegia
   C. Enlargement of extraocular muscles
   D. Lid lag.

18. Dalrymple sign is seen in:
   A. Thyroid ophthalmopathy
   B. Cavernous sinus thrombosis
   C. Orbital cellulitis
   D. Cavernous haemangioma.

19. First muscle to be involved in thyroid ophthalmopathy is:
   A. Medial rectus
   B. Inferior rectus
   C. Lateral rectus
   D. Superior rectus.

20. Thyroid ophthalmopathy: All of the following are treatment modalities except:
   A. Radiation
   B. Steroids
   C. B-Blockers
   D. Orbital decompression.

21. Which is a pathognomonic CT Finding in Thyroid ophthalmopathy?
   A. Kinking of extraocular muscles
   B. Nodular muscle enlargement
   C. Fusiform muscle enlargement with sparing of tendons
   D. Solitary muscle enlargement.

22. Which is the commonest eyelid finding in Thyroid ophthalmopathy?
   A. Lid lag
   B. Lagophthalmos
   C. Lid retaction
   D. Von Graefe's sign.

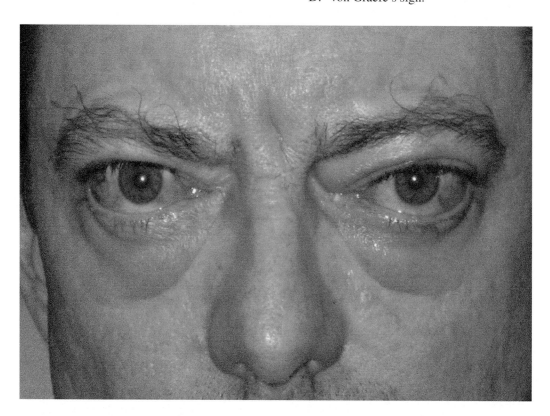

23. A 55-year-old white man presents with bilateral proptosis, double vision, and chemosis. What is the most likely diagnosis?

    A. Thyroid-related orbitopathy
    B. Orbital cellulitis
    C. Lymphangioma
    D. Meningioma.

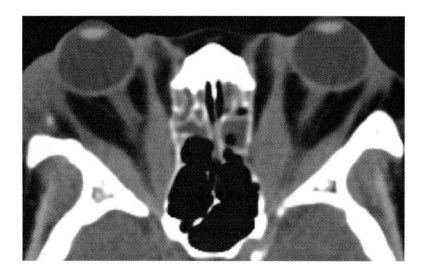

24. A CT is performed on this patient with thyroid orbitopathy. Which feature, as demonstrated by CT, helps to clarify that this process is more likely thyroid-related orbitopathy than orbital inflammatory syndrome?
    A. Enlarged extraocular muscle
    B. Absence of a thickened tendon of the extraocular muscle insertion
    C. Enlarged lacrimal glands
    D. Periorbital soft-tissue edema of the lids.

25. Which of the following CT findings is not commonly seen with thyroid-related orbitopathy?
    A. Sparing of extraocular muscle tendons
    B. Involvement of extraocular muscle tendons

    C. Fusiform extraocular muscle involvement
    D. Bilateral extraocular muscle involvement.

26. What are the 2 most commonly affected rectus muscles in thyroid eye disease?
    A. Superior and inferior
    B. Superior and medial
    C. Medial and lateral
    D. Inferior and medial.

27. Which condition is closely associated with thyroid eye disease?
    A. Eczematous eyelid
    B. Parinaud's syndrome
    C. Myotonic dystrophy
    D. Myasthenia gravis.

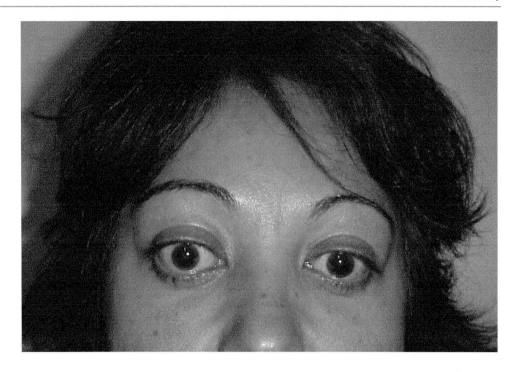

28. The patient is looking down, this is called:
    A. Lagophthalmos
    B. Lid lag
    C. Lid retraction
    D. Von Graefe's sign.

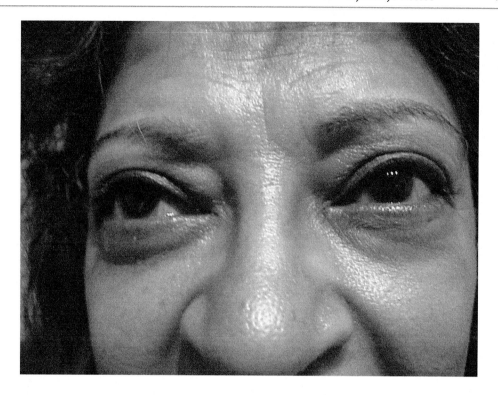

29. This Thyroid patient requires:
    A. Lid retraction surgery
    B. Strabismus surgery
    C. Blepharoplasty
    D. Spacer.

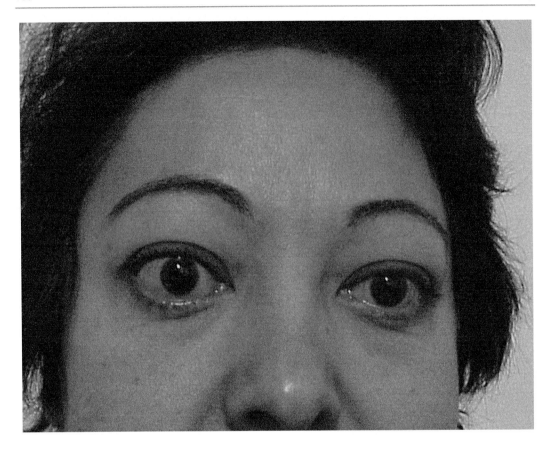

30. This patient requires:
    A. Lid retraction surgery
    B. Strabismus surgery
    C. Blepharoplasty
    D. Spacer.

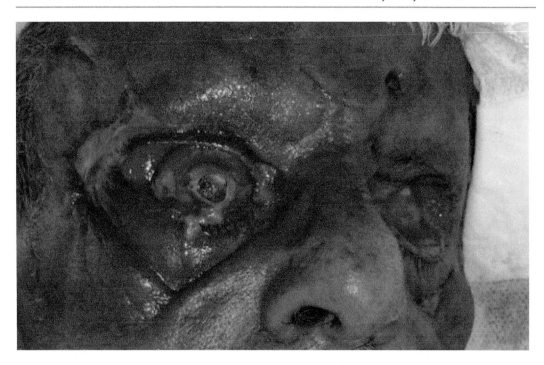

31. In thyroid ophthalmopathy, this is a compli-
    cation of all except:
    A. Severe proptosis

    B. Corneal exposure
    C. Optic nerve compression
    D. Improper Streroid therapy.

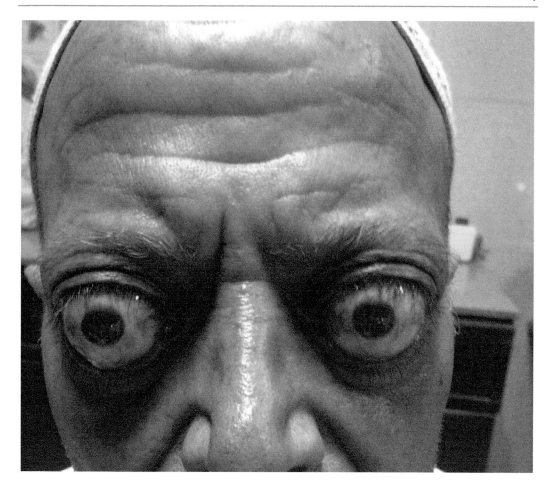

32. This Thyroid patient requires:
    A. Lid retraction surgery
    B. Decompression surgery
    C. Blepharoplasty
    D. IV steroid therapy.

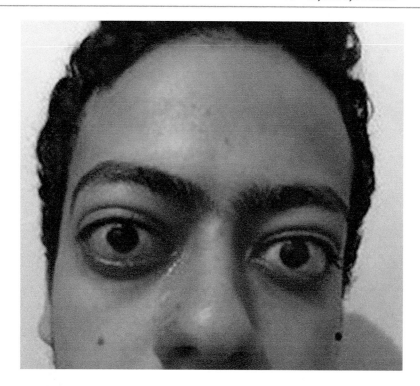

33. This young patient will most likely benefit from;
    A. Decompression
    B. IV steroids
    C. Intraorbital steroids
    D. Radiation.

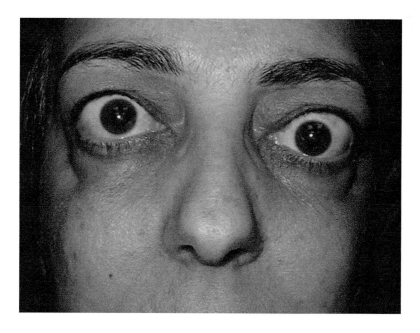

34. This patient will benefit from:
    A. Lid retraction surgery
    B. Decompression surgery
    C. Blepharoplasty
    D. IV steroid therapy.

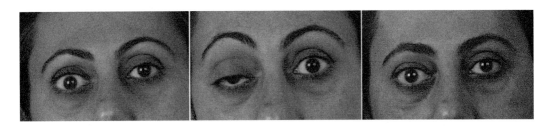

35. This appearance in a thyroid patient suggests;
    A. Noncompliance with medication
    B. Myasthenia gravis

C. Steroid resistance
D. Severe levator muscle affection.

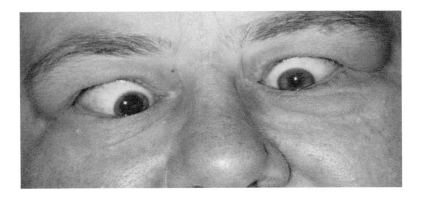

36. This is a complication of:
    A. Inferior wall decompression
    B. Medial wall decompression
    C. Two wall decompression
    D. Balanced decompression.
37. All the following injections can be used in Thyroid ophthalmopathy except:
    A. Botulinium toxin
    B. Steroids

C. B-blockers
D. Fillers.
38. Promising results for the treatment of thyroid ophthalmopathy has been achieved with the use of:
    A. Ranibizumab
    B. Bevacizumab
    C. Teprotumumab
    D. Rituximab.

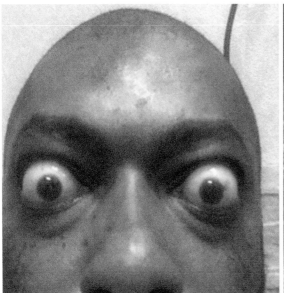
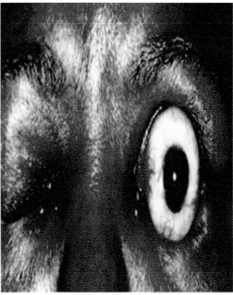

39. This complication occurs due to:
    A. Proptosis
    B. Lid retraction
    C. Proptosis and lid retraction
    D. Increased orbital pressure.

40. Rundle's curve in thyroid ophthalmopathy describes:
    A. Disease pathology
    B. Disease activity
    C. Disease prognosis
    D. Disease management.

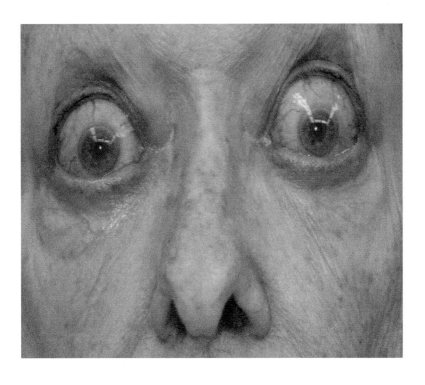

41. Management of this patient requires:
    A. Lid retraction surgery
    B. Decompression surgery
    C. Blepharoplasty
    D. IV steroid therapy.

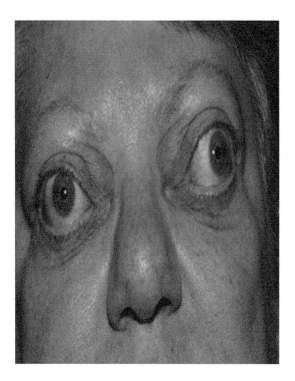 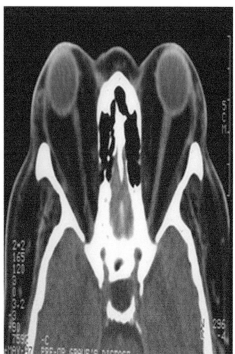

42. This patient has:
    A. Type 1 thyroid ophthalmopathy
    B. Type 2 thyroid ophthalmopathy
    C. A CAS score of 5
    D. Mild disease by the EUGOGO scale.

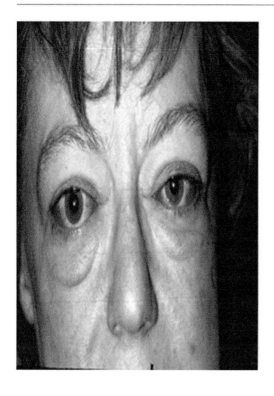

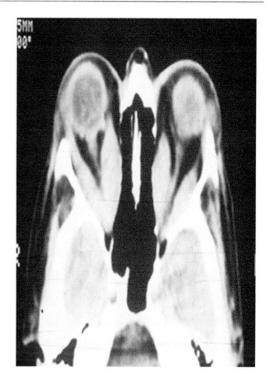

43. This patient has:
    A. Type 1 thyroid ophthalmopathy
    B. Type 2 thyroid ophthalmopathy
    C. A CAS score of 5
    D. Mild disease by the EUGOGO scale.

44. The CAS score has:
    A. 5 points
    B. 7 points
    C. 8 points
    D. 10 points.

45. The EUGOGO scale has:
    A. 2 grades
    B. 3 grades
    C. 4 grades
    D. 5 grades.

46. Balanaced decompression means removal of:
    A. Parts of medial wall and inferior wall
    B. Parts of medial wall and lateral wall
    C. Parts of lateral wall and inferior wall
    D. Equal parts of all three walls.

47. Inferior decompression can be done through all except:
    A. Transcutaneous approach
    B. Transconjunctival approach
    C. Transantral approach
    D. Transnasal approach.

48. Medial decompression can be done through all except:
    A. Transcutaneous approach
    B. Transantral approach
    C. Transcaruncular approach
    D. Transnasal approach.

49. Lateral decompression can be done through:
    A. Transcutaneous approach
    B. Transconjunctival approach
    C. Transcaruncular approach
    D. Transnasal approach.

50. Advantages of intraorbital steroids in the active phase of thyroid ophthalmopathy include all except:
    A. No or lower doses of systemic steroids
    B. Single injection is sufficient
    C. Improves lid retraction
    D. Reduces incidence of recurrence.

51. Corticosteroids are used in treatment of all except;
    A. Orbital lymphoma

B. Thyroid eye disease
C. Orbital mucocele
D. Non specific orbital inflammation.

52. Limitation of ocular motility occurs in all except
    A. Orbital rim fracture
    B. Cavernous sinus thrombosis
    C. Orbital cellulitis
    D. Thyroid orbitopathy.

53. Which of the following is the recommended management of dysthyroid optic neuropathy (DON)?
    A. Intravenous steroid
    B. Oral steroid
    C. Radiotherapy
    D. Selenium.

54. Which of the following is the best indicator of activity in thyroid eye disease?
    A. Diplopia
    B. Upper lid edema
    C. Pain
    D. Reduced color vision.

Answers for Thyroid Eye Disease

1	D	16	C	31	C	46	B
2	D	17	B	32	B	47	D
3	D	18	A	33	C	48	B
4	B	19	B	34	A	49	A
5	C	20	C	35	B	50	B
6	C	21	C	36	A	51	C
7	A	22	C	37	C	52	A
8	B	23	A	38	C	53	A
9	B	24	B	39	C	54	B
10	B	25	B	40	B		
11	A	26	D	41	B		
12	A	27	D	42	A		
13	C	28	B	43	B		
14	C	29	C	44	D		
15	A	30	A	45	B		

Printed in the United States
by Baker & Taylor Publisher Services